Pancreatitis

Edited by Dmitry Victorovich Garbuzenko

Published in London, United Kingdom

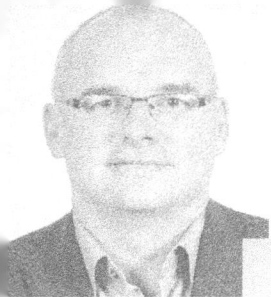
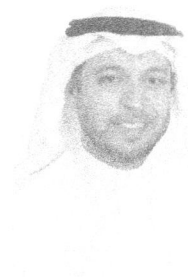
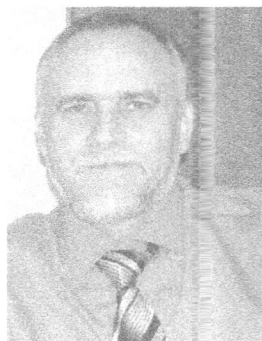
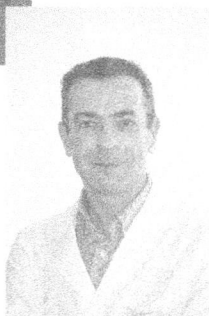
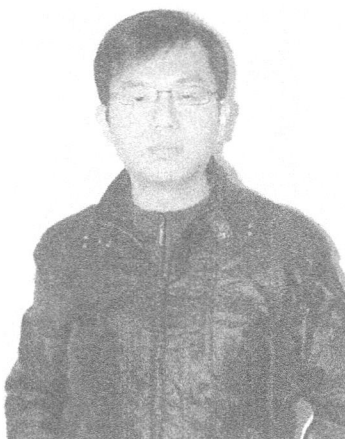
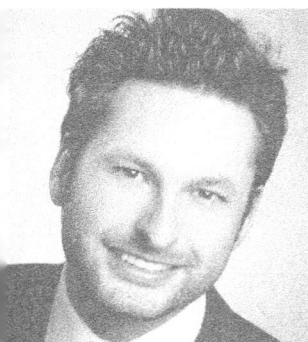
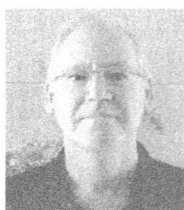

IntechOpen

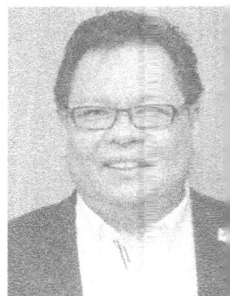
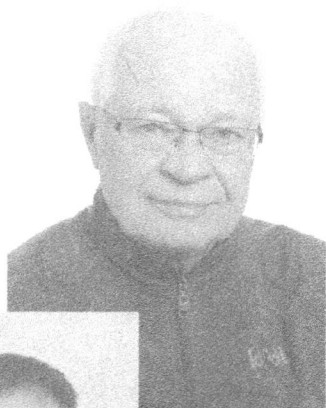
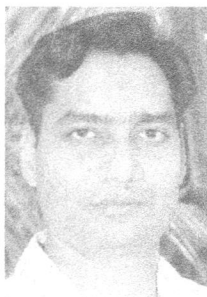
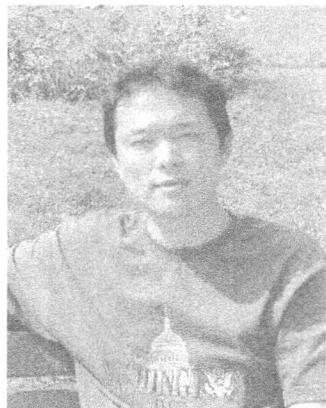
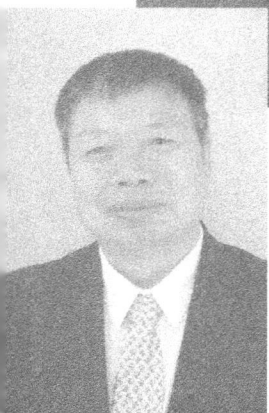
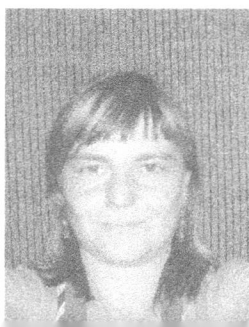

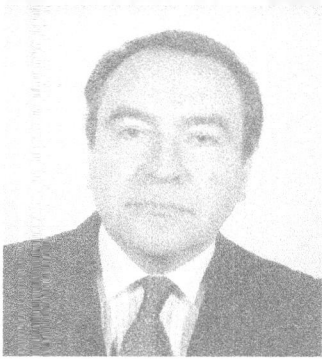

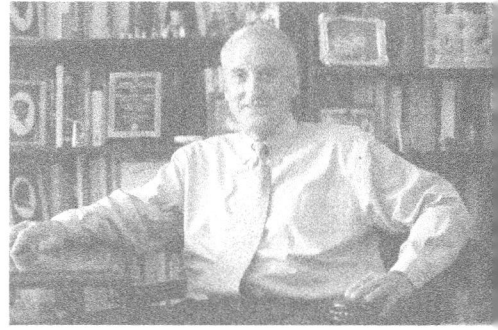

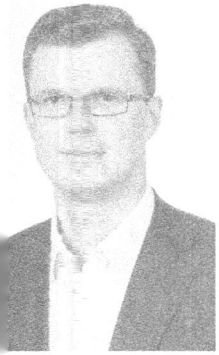

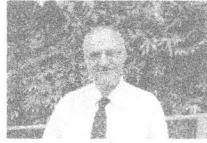

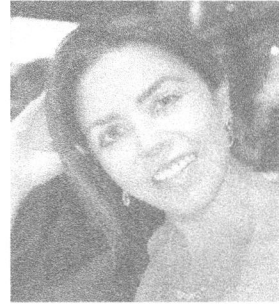

Supporting open minds since 2005

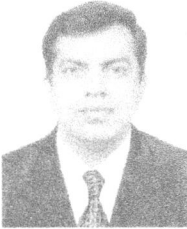

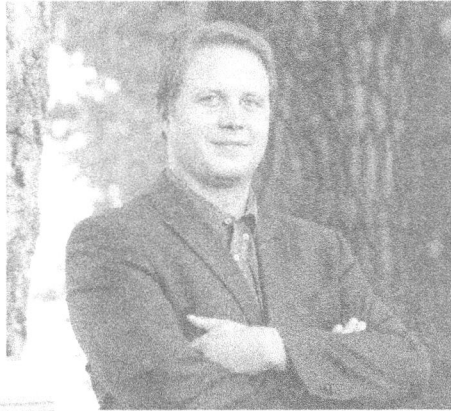

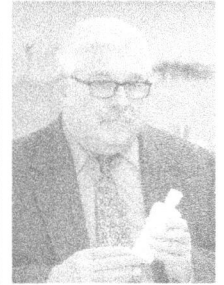

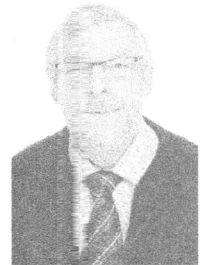

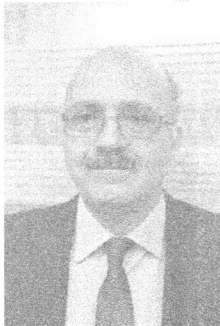

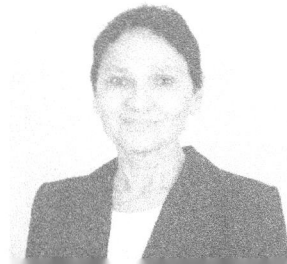

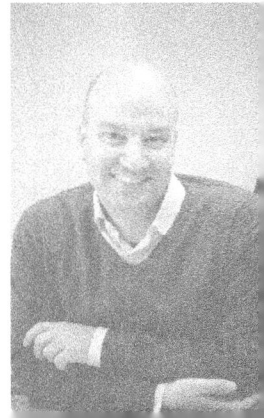

Pancreatitis
http://dx.doi.org/10.5772/intechopen.77681
Edited by Dmitry Victorovich Garbuzenko

Contributors
Mila Dimitrova Kovacheva-Slavova, Borislav Vladimirov, Plamen Gecov, Georgi Vladimirov, Stefano Valabrega, Laura Bersigotti, Luciano Izzo, Federico Tomassini, Laura Antolino, Salvatore Caterino, Paolo Aurello, Francesco D'Angelo, Cosmas Rinaldi A Lesmana, Laurentius Lesmana, Khek Yu Ho, Zaheer Nabi, Dmitry Victorovich Garbuzenko

Notice
Statements and opinions expressed in the chapters are these of the individual contributors and not necessarily those of the editors or publisher. No responsibility is accepted for the accuracy of information contained in the published chapters. The publisher assumes no responsibility for any damage or injury to persons or property arising out of the use of any materials, instructions, methods or ideas contained in the book.

First published in London, United Kingdom, 2019 by IntechOpen
IntechOpen is the global imprint of INTECHOPEN LIMITED, registered in England and Wales, registration number: 11086078, 7th floor, 10 Lower Thames Street, London, EC3R 6AF, United Kingdom
Printed in Croatia

British Library Cataloguing-in-Publication Data
A catalogue record for this book is available from the British Library

Additional hard and PDF copies can be obtained from orders@intechopen.com

Pancreatitis
Edited by Dmitry Victorovich Garbuzenko
p. cm.
Print ISBN 978-1-83968-149-3
Online ISBN 978-1-83968-150-9
eBook (PDF) ISBN 978-1-83968-151-6

We are IntechOpen,
the world's leading publisher of
Open Access books
Built by scientists, for scientists

4,500+
Open access books available

118,000+
International authors and editors

130M+
Downloads

Our authors are among the

151
Countries delivered to

Top 1%
most cited scientists

12.2%
Contributors from top 500 universities

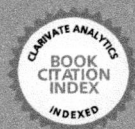

Interested in publishing with us?
Contact book.department@intechopen.com

Numbers displayed above are based on latest data collected.
For more information visit www.intechopen.com

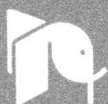

Meet the editor

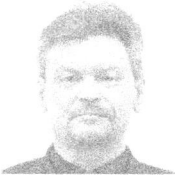

Dmitry Victorovich Garbuzenko graduated from the Chelyabinsk State Medical Institute in 1985. From 1985 to 1987, he was a clinical intern. From 1987 to 1990, he was a post-graduate student at the Hospital Surgery Department in Chelyabinsk State Medical Academy. In 1991, he defended his Ph.D. thesis. He was an assistant in the Department of Hospital Surgery from 1991 to 1996. In 1996, he became an Assistant, and then an Associate Professor (2003), and then Professor (2006) of the Department of Faculty Surgery, South Ural State Medical University. In 2008, he defended his doctoral thesis (M.D.). Professor Garbuzenko is a member of the Russian Society of Surgeons. His practical activities focus on emergency abdominal surgery. He is the author of nearly 170 publications.

Contents

Preface

The book "Pancreatitis" is devoted to the actual and, in some cases, controversial and unresolved problems associated with acute and chronic pancreatitis. Acute pancreatitis is one of the most common causes of acute abdomen. Along with an increase in the number of patients with acute pancreatitis in recent years, there has been an increase in the incidence of its destructive forms. Despite the progress in improving the diagnostics of the disease, pathogenetically substantiated intensive therapy, antibiotic therapy, and minimally invasive surgical treatment, mortality in acute pancreatitis has remained at the same level over the past few decades. The most important objective in improving treatment results in acute pancreatitis is the use of standardized approaches to diagnostics and treatment of various forms of the disease and its complications, taking into account the modern, generally accepted international classification. Chronic pancreatitis is characterized by inflammation of the pancreas, which is replaced by fibrosis and progressing pancreatic tissue destruction. The three main clinical signs of chronic pancreatitis are pain, maldigestion, and diabetes. Although the disease is still difficult to treat, the development of new approaches has reduced the severity of clinical manifestations and improved the life quality of patients with chronic pancreatitis. This book will be of interest to anyone who considers pancreatology their specialty.

Dmitry Victorovich Garbuzenko
Professor,
Department of Faculty Surgery,
South Ural State Medical University,
Chelyabinsk, Russia

Introductory Chapter: Current Challenges in the Management of Patients with Acute and Chronic Pancreatitis

Dmitry Garbuzenko

1. Introduction

As part of medical science, pancreatology reflects the level of technological progress and modern achievements in the natural sciences. Over the past five centuries, since A. Vesalius first described the pancreas and its topography, tremendous work has been done to determine the physiological role of the pancreas in the process of digestion, to study the causes and patterns characteristic of pancreatic diseases, and to find the ways of treatment. In this regard, the current challenges in modern pancreatology include the development and implementation of methods for early and accurate diagnosis and selection of the optimal tactics for treating patients with acute and chronic pancreatitis.

2. Acute pancreatitis

Acute pancreatitis is an acute surgical disease of the pancreas, which consists of primary edema or aseptic necrosis of pancreatic parenchyma with the possible infection of the pancreas and retroperitoneal tissue. Acute pancreatitis is one of the most common causes of acute abdomen, ranking third after acute appendicitis and acute cholecystitis. Along with an increase in the number of patients with acute pancreatitis in recent years, there has been a tendency to an increase in the incidence of its destructive forms [1].

Despite the progress achieved in improving the diagnostics of acute pancreatitis, pathogenetically substantiated intensive therapy, antibiotic therapy, and minimally invasive surgical treatment, mortality in acute pancreatitis has remained at the same level over the past decades. Moreover, while the overall mortality is within 3–6%, depending on the fluctuation of destructive pancreatitis incidence, the mortality rate is 15–30% in pancreatic necrosis, is 85% in infected pancreatic necrosis, and reaches 100% in fulminant acute pancreatitis [2].

Currently, the immediate prescription of antibiotics in severe forms of acute pancreatitis is no longer debatable. However, there are still different opinions on the effectiveness of existing methods of delivering antibacterial drugs to the site of pancreatic destruction. The situation is aggravated by the increasing polyresistance of microorganisms to most antimicrobial chemotherapeutic agents [3]. According to modern conception, immune disorders are considered as a factor that largely determines the course of acute pancreatitis, helps maintain the inflammatory process, and reduces the effectiveness of reparative mechanisms [4]. In this regard, an urgent problem is the early prevention of infection in severe pancreatitis, timely detection and correction of immunological deficiency, and timely diagnosis and treatment of septic complications including systemic inflammatory response, multiple organ failure, and sepsis [5].

At present, some certainty has been achieved in approaches to the management of patients with acute pancreatitis. Nevertheless, one of the most important problems is to choose the tactics of surgical treatment. Mild pancreatitis does not require surgery and quickly disappears after using standard conservative treatment and eliminating the etiological factor. However, in 10–20% of patients, surgeons encounter severe pancreatic necrosis, which is essentially a hypermetabolic syndrome of multiple organ failure. While the questions about the indications and the most favorable time period for surgical treatment are mostly answered in severe pancreatitis, it is still not obvious what the most appropriate techniques and type of surgery are. Along with experience in minimally invasive interventions, it becomes clear that their active implementation does not solve all the problems of acute pancreatitis treatment and requires further research [6].

Thus, the most important objective in improving treatment results in acute pancreatitis is the use of standardized approaches to diagnostics and treatment of various forms of the disease and its complications, taking into account the modern generally accepted international classification [7].

3. Chronic pancreatitis

Chronic pancreatitis is characterized by inflammation of the pancreas, which is replaced by fibrosis and progressing pancreatic tissue destruction. According to the M-ANNHEIM classification, the following etiological causes are involved in the pathogenesis of chronic pancreatitis: alcohol consumption, nicotine consumption, nutrition factors, hereditary factors, efferent duct factors, immunological risk factors, and miscellaneous (tropical chronic pancreatitis, primary hypercalcemia, hyperparathyroidism, hyperlipidemia) [8]. Clinically, at an early stage of the disease, abdominal pain or recurrent episodes of acute pancreatitis usually prevail, whereas, at a late stage, symptoms are associated with exocrine and/or endocrine insufficiency. Consequently, the three main clinical signs of chronic pancreatitis are pain, maldigestion, and diabetes. The incidence is estimated at 2–10/100000 and tends to increase [9]. In addition, there are many patients with characteristic symptoms but with undiagnosed chronic pancreatitis.

Chronic pancreatitis is not only an urgent medical problem but also a significant economic burden that has a profound effect on social life and the structure of employment [10]. In the United States in 2000, there were 327,000 hospitalizations and 532,000 visits to doctors due to chronic pancreatitis, which cost $2.5 billion [11].

Diagnostics and follow-up of patients with chronic pancreatitis are based on both the clinical picture and imaging methods, and the diagnosis of chronic pancreatitis at an early stage is a clinical problem. Historically, diagnostic methods included ultrasound imaging of the abdominal organs, endoscopic ultrasound (EUS), ultrasound with contrast enhancement (CEUS), endoscopic retrograde cholangiopancreatography (ERCP), magnetic resonance imaging (MRI), and computed tomography (CT). While ultrasound is considered the least accurate, and EUS is one of the most sensitive methods [12], ERCP is no longer a diagnostic test for chronic pancreatitis [13]. EUS is highly accurate in assessing the parenchyma and ductal system of the pancreas and is also very useful in identifying complication characteristic of chronic pancreatitis [14]. CEUS helps diagnose cystic and solid lesions of the pancreas, which are associated with chronic pancreatitis. It was convincing in 90% of cases, so it may be considered as a first-line method of visualization [15]. MRI makes it possible to accurately determine the morphological and functional changes of the pancreas and is a recognized method for detecting calculi in pancreatic ducts [16]. At the same time, the calcinates may be determined by means of portal-phase contrast-enhanced CT with moderate sensitivity and very high specificity (close to 100%) [17].

The degree of exocrine and endocrine pancreatic insufficiency is also important to determine when diagnosing chronic pancreatitis. The so-called direct or invasive methods for detecting exocrine insufficiency, such as the Lund test, are a thing of the past. Currently, the "gold standard" is 3-day fecal fat quantification and determination of the coefficient of fat absorption. Due to the cumbersomeness and unpleasantness of the method for both patient and laboratory personnel, it is very rarely used in everyday clinical practice. Other methods for diagnosing exocrine pancreatic insufficiency include measuring the concentration of fecal elastase 1, the ^{13}C-mixed triglycerides (^{13}C-MTG) breath test, a test based on analysis of pancreatic juice after secretin/cerulein stimulation, and others [18].

In the absence of complications, the main goal of treating chronic pancreatitis is the effective correction of its main manifestations: pain, maldigestion, and diabetes. Abdominal pain is usually severe and often occurs after a meal, which, despite adequate enzyme replacement therapy, leads to malnutrition. Although pain may be associated with strictures and stones in the main pancreatic duct, new investigations have questioned the importance of micro- and macrostructural pathological changes. Currently, the neurogenic causes of pain are widely discussed, which should be taken into account when choosing the method of pain relief for patients [19]. Malnutrition that is related to a lack of enzymes leads not only to weight loss but also to a certain deficiency of vitamins and nutrients that are necessary for normal physiological functioning. Malnutrition in chronic pancreatitis is often overlooked. It is very important that gastroenterologists consider this fact while making a differential diagnosis in patients with weight loss [20]. Diabetes of the exocrine pancreas is a form of diabetes that occurs due to pancreatic disease. It is more common than previously thought. A recent study found that in 1.8% of adults with diabetes, it should be classified as diabetes of the exocrine pancreas. However, in most cases, it is referred to as type 2 diabetes. Patients with diabetes of the exocrine pancreas have varying degrees of exocrine and endocrine dysfunction. Damage to the islets of Langerhans affects the secretion of hormones by the pancreatic polypeptide, β-, and α-cells. Polypeptides and a low concentration of insulin and glucagon promote sharp fluctuations in the glucose level. This form of "fragile diabetes" in patients with diabetes of the exocrine pancreas may lead to worse glycemic control in comparison with type 2 diabetes [21].

If conservative therapy is not effective, it is possible to apply the endoscopic treatment, conduction anesthesia or neurolysis, or surgical techniques. Endoscopic methods are usually required for the elimination of the main pancreatic duct obstruction caused by a stricture or stone. In addition, endoscopy is the first-choice treatment of pancreatic pseudocysts [22]. Celiac plexus block is useful for eliminating pain. It is performed via a gastric approach using EUS guidance and has high success rates and relatively low complication rates [23]. Surgical treatment of chronic pancreatitis is aimed primarily at relieving pain, improving the patient's quality of life, and treating complications. Surgical operations include decompression (drainage) of the main pancreatic duct, various types of pancreatic resections, their combination, and neuroablation [24].

In recent years, important advances have been made in understanding the pathogenesis of chronic pancreatitis. Although the disease is still difficult to treat, the development of new approaches has reduced the severity of clinical manifestations and improved the life quality of patients with chronic pancreatitis.

Author details

Dmitry Garbuzenko
Department of Faculty Surgery, South Ural State Medical University, Chelyabinsk, Russia

*Address all correspondence to: garb@inbox.ru

IntechOpen

References

[1] Garbuzenko DV. Selected Lectures in Emergency Abdominal Surgery. Saarbrücken, Germany: LAP LAMBERT Academic Publishing GmbH and Co; 2012

[2] Karakayali FY. Surgical and interventional management of complications caused by acute pancreatitis. World Journal of Gastroenterology. 2014;**20**(37):13412-13423

[3] Ukai T, Shikata S, Inoue M, Noguchi Y, Igarashi H, Isaji S, et al. Early prophylactic antibiotics administration for acute necrotizing pancreatitis: A meta-analysis of randomized controlled trials. Journal of Hepato-Biliary-Pancreatic Sciences. 2015;**22**(4):316-321

[4] Li J, Yang WJ, Huang LM, Tang CW. Immunomodulatory therapies for acute pancreatitis. World Journal of Gastroenterology. 2014;**20**(45):16935-16947

[5] Mourad MM, Evans R, Kalidindi V, Navaratnam R, Dvorkin L, Bramhall SR. Prophylactic antibiotics in acute pancreatitis: Endless debate. Annals of the Royal College of Surgeons of England. 2017;**99**(2):107-112

[6] Kokosis G, Perez A, Pappas TN. Surgical management of necrotizing pancreatitis: An overview. World Journal of Gastroenterology. 2014;**20**(43):16106-16112

[7] Crockett SD, Wani S, Gardner TB, Falck-Ytter Y, Barkun AN, American Gastroenterological Association Institute Clinical Guidelines Committee. American Gastroenterological Association Institute Guideline on initial management of acute pancreatitis. Gastroenterology. 2018;**154**(4):1096-1101

[8] Brock C, Nielsen LM, Lelic D, Drewes AM. Pathophysiology of chronic pancreatitis. World Journal of Gastroenterology. 2013;**19**(42):7231-7240

[9] Yadav D, Timmons L, Benson JT, Dierkhising RA, Chari ST. Incidence, prevalence, and survival of chronic pancreatitis: A population-based study. The American Journal of Gastroenterology. 2011;**106**(12):2192-2199

[10] Gardner TB, Kennedy AT, Gelrud A, Banks PA, Vege SS, Gordon SR, et al. Chronic pancreatitis and its effect on employment and health care experience: Results of a prospective American multicenter study. Pancreas. 2010;**39**(4):498-501

[11] Lowenfels AB, Sullivan T, Fiorianti J, Maisonneuve P. The epidemiology and impact of pancreatic diseases in the United States. Current Gastroenterology Reports. 2005;7(2):90-95

[12] Löhr JM, Dominguez-Munoz E, Rosendahl J, Besselink M, Mayerle J, Lerch MM, et al. United European gastroenterology evidence-based guidelines for the diagnosis and therapy of chronic pancreatitis (HaPanEU). United European Gastroenterology Journal. 2017;**5**(2):153-199

[13] Iglesias-García J, Lariño-Noia J, Lindkvist B, Domínguez-Muñoz JE. Endoscopic ultrasound in the diagnosis of chronic pancreatitis. Revista Española de Enfermedades Digestivas. 2015;**107**(4):221-228

[14] Iglesias-García J, Lindkvist B, Lariño-Noia J, Domínguez-Muñoz JE. The role of EUS in relation to other imaging modalities in the differential diagnosis between mass forming chronic pancreatitis, autoimmune pancreatitis and ductal pancreatic adenocarcinoma.

Revista Española de Enfermedades Digestivas. 2012;**104**(6):315-321

[15] Ardelean M, Şirli R, Sporea I, Bota S, Martie A, Popescu A, et al. Contrast enhanced ultrasound in the pathology of the pancreas—A monocentric experience. Medical Ultrasonography. 2014;**16**(4):325-331

[16] Hansen TM, Nilsson M, Gram M, Frøkjær JB. Morphological and functional evaluation of chronic pancreatitis with magnetic resonance imaging. World Journal of Gastroenterology. 2013;**19**(42):7241-7246

[17] Anderson SW, Soto JA. Pancreatic duct evaluation: Accuracy of portal venous phase 64 MDCT. Abdominal Imaging. 2009;**34**(1):55-63

[18] Dominguez-Muñoz JE. Diagnosis and treatment of pancreatic exocrine insufficiency. Current Opinion in Gastroenterology. 2018;**34**(5):349-354

[19] Olesen SS, Juel J, Graversen C, Kolesnikov Y, Wilder-Smith OH, Drewes AM. Pharmacological pain management in chronic pancreatitis. World Journal of Gastroenterology. 2013;**19**(42):7292-7301

[20] Rasmussen HH, Irtun O, Olesen SS, Drewes AM, Holst M. Nutrition in chronic pancreatitis. World Journal of Gastroenterology. 2013;**19**(42):7267-7275

[21] Wynne K, Devereaux B, Dornhorst A. Diabetes of the exocrine pancreas. Journal of Gastroenterology and Hepatology. 2019;**34**(2):346-354

[22] Oza VM, Kahaleh M. Endoscopic management of chronic pancreatitis. World Journal of Gastrointestinal Endoscopy. 2013;**5**(1):19-28

[23] Gress F, Schmitt C, Sherman S, Ciaccia D, Ikenberry S, Lehman G. Endoscopic ultrasound-guided celiac plexus block for managing abdominal pain associated with chronic pancreatitis: A prospective single center experience. The American Journal of Gastroenterology. 2001;**96**(2):409-416

[24] Ni Q, Yun L, Roy M, Shang D. Advances in surgical treatment of chronic pancreatitis. World Journal of Surgical Oncology. 2015;**13**:34

Chapter 2

Endoscopic Management of Pancreatic Fluid Collections: An Update

Zaheer Nabi and D. Nageshwar Reddy

Abstract

Pancreatic fluid collections (PFCs) are a frequent complication of acute pancreatitis. PFCs have been categorized according to their content and duration after an episode of pancreatitis. Acute collections (<4 week) and asymptomatic late collections (>4 weeks) can be usually managed conservatively. Late collections including walled off necrosis (WON) and pancreatic pseudocysts (PP) have a well-defined wall. Consequently, it is easier and safer to drain these collections when required. The most common indication to drain PFCs is infection and the available means of drainage include surgical, endoscopic, and percutaneous. Open surgical interventions carry a high risk of morbidity and mortality. Therefore, in the current era, a step up approach is preferred to minimize morbidity over the more aggressive surgical treatments. Endoscopic step-up approach is effective and favored over minimally invasive surgical or percutaneous drainage due to reduced risk of organ failure and external pancreatic fistula. However, the approach to PFCs should be individualized for optimal outcomes. A small subgroup of patients does not respond to endotherapy or percutaneous interventions and requires open surgical debridement. Similarly, not all PFCs are amenable to endoscopic drainage and demand alternative modalities like percutaneous or minimally invasive surgical drainage.

Keywords: pancreatitis, pseudocyst, walled off necrosis, drainage, endoscopy

1. Introduction

Acute pancreatitis is mild in majority of the cases and categorized as interstitial edematous pancreatitis. About 15–20% of cases develop necrotizing pancreatitis involving necrosis of variable proportion of pancreatic parenchyma. Pancreatic fluid collections (PFCs) are a common local complication of acute pancreatitis. PFCs have been classified according to the revised Atlanta criteria based on duration (<4 or >4 weeks) and contents of fluid collection [1]. Acute collections include acute pancreatic or peri-pancreatic fluid collections (APFCs) and acute necrotic pancreatic fluid collections (ANPFCs) which develop after acute interstitial and acute necrotizing pancreatitis, respectively (**Figure 1**). APFCs and ANPFCs get walled off after about 4–6 weeks into pseudocysts and walled off necrosis (WON), respectively. By definition, pseudocysts have clear contents and WON consists of variable amount of necrotic debris (**Figures 2** and **3**).

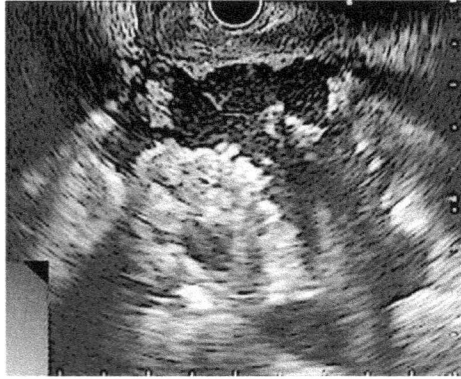

Figure 1.
Endosonographic image of acute necrotic pancreatic fluid collections. Note the ill-defined boundaries and the solid component within the fluid collection.

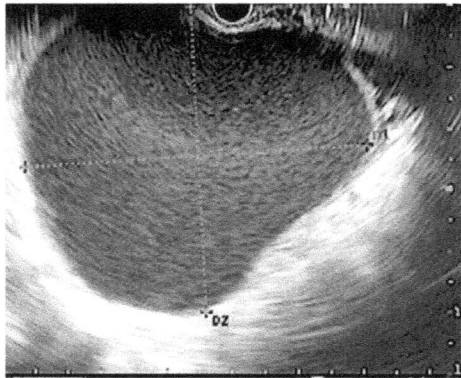

Figure 2.
Endosonographic image in a case with pancreatic pseudocyst. Not the well-defined boundaries without any echogenic debris in the cyst cavity.

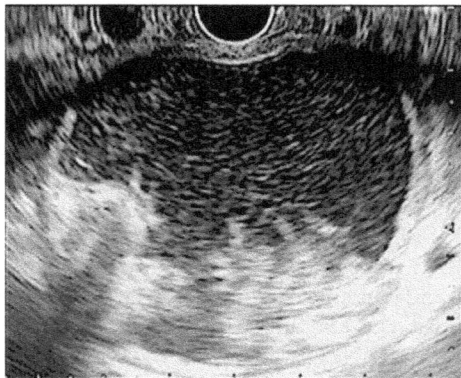

Figure 3.
Endosonographic image in a case with walled off necrosis. Not the well-defined boundaries with echogenic necrotic debris in the cyst cavity.

1.1 Natural history of pancreatic fluid collections

APFCs develop in about 20–40% of patients after acute interstitial pancreatitis [2–4]. Majority (~90%) of APFCs resolve and do not transform into pseudocyst. Moreover, majority of the pseudocysts resolve or reduce in size with time and therefore, do not require an intervention [4]. On the other hand, majority (90–100%) of the patients with acute necrotizing pancreatitis develop ANPFCs. Nearly half of the patients with ANPFCs develop walled off necrosis (WON) [2, 3]. The natural history of WON is not well known and appears to be more unpredictable than pseudocysts. An intervention may be required in one quarter to more than half of the patients with WON [2, 3].

2. Management of pancreatic fluid collections

The options of drainage for PFCs include surgery, percutaneous catheter drainage, and endoscopic transmural drainage (ETD). Open necrosectomy is associated with substantial rates of new onset multiple organ failure as compared to minimally invasive surgical step up approach (see later) [5]. Subsequent studies comparing endoscopic necrosectomy to open as well as minimally invasive surgical debridement concluded the superiority of endoscopic approach [6, 7]. Reduced mortality, less frequent new onset multiple organ failure, and the development of pancreatic fistulas are distinct advantages of endoscopic necrosectomy [8, 9]. In the current era, a step up approach is preferred for its obvious benefits in reducing a pro-inflammatory response and prevention of new onset organ failure. In the ensuing sections, we would discuss endoscopic approach to PFCs and its advantages over surgical and percutaneous drainages.

2.1 Endoscopic drainage of PFCs

Characterization of PFCs into pseudocysts and WON is important prior to ETD. WON has variable amount of necrotic debris and therefore, has a protracted course and more frequent requirement of re-interventions as compared to pseudocysts (**Figures 2** and **3**). Computed tomography is frequently used to localize the site of collection. However, it may not accurately differentiate between the solid and liquid contents of the collection (**Figures 4** and **5**). Magnetic resonance imaging (MRI)

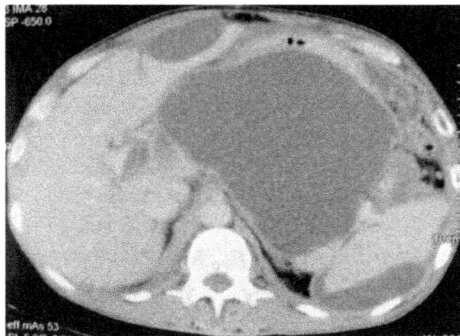

Figure 4.
CT image in a case of pancreatic pseudocyst. Note the well-defined boundary and clear contents of the cyst.

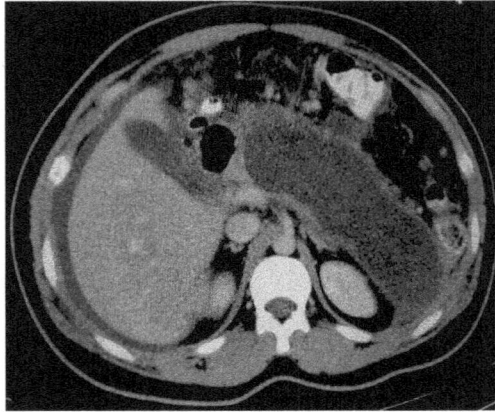

Figure 5.
CT image in a case of walled off necrosis replacing almost entire pancreas. Note that the necrotic contents of the cyst cavity are not obvious in CT image.

and endoscopic ultrasound (EUS) are better imaging modalities for qualitative assessment of PFCs. We perform both CECT and EUS to define the anatomical relation of PFCs to the lumen and characterize them into pseudocyst or WON, respectively.

The technique of endoscopic drainage of PFCs involves the following steps: puncture of the cysto-gastric or cysto-duodenal wall using a 19 gauge needle and aspiration of cyst contents, coiling of guidewire within the cyst cavity under fluoroscopy guidance, dilatation of the tract using cystotome and balloon and deployment of plastic or metal endoprostheses. EUS guided drainage is preferred to endoscopic approach as intervening vessels can be avoided and non-bulging collections can be targeted under vision [10].

The success rate of ETD with or without endoscopic necrosectomy ranges from 80 to 95% in recent studies [11–19] (**Table 1**). The outcomes of ETD of PFCs is variable in literature presumably due to heterogeneity in the nature of collection, that is, pseudocyst or WON, type of stent used, and whether necrosectomy is performed or not [20]. In addition, the presence of disconnected pancreatic duct (DPD) may impact the outcomes of ETD. The requirement of hybrid treatment, re-interventions, recurrences, and rescue surgery appear to be higher in the patients with DPD [21].

ETD of PFCs is safe, and major complications are uncommon. Complications related to ETD occur in 10–40% of patients with WON [22]. Supra-infection of the cyst cavity is the most common significant complication associated with ETD. Occlusion of the stent with necrotic debris and inadequate drainage may lead to sepsis. In such situations, de-clogging of the metal stent, cyst lavage with saline or diluted hydrogen peroxide and direct endoscopic necrosectomy (DEN) are often helpful. Other complications associated with ETD include bleeding and perforation. Recent studies have drawn attention towards the relatively high incidence of bleeding especially with the use of large caliber metal stents (LCMS) [23–25]. Since, majority of the bleeding episodes occurred ≥3 weeks after the deployment of LCMS, the current trend is to remove LCMS between 2 and 3 weeks in cases of resolution of PFC [24].

2.2 Endoscopic transmural drainage: choice of stents

Endoscopic drainage of PFCs can be performed using pigtail plastic stents or metal stents. Plastic stents have been effectively used for the drainage of PFCs for

	N	PFC	Type of stent	Success	Recurrence	Adjuvant PCD or Sx	Complications
Walter et al. [11]	61	PC 15 WON 46	LAMS (AXIOS)	93% 81%	NR	Sx 6.5%	Infection 6.5% Perforation 1.6%
Siddiqui et al. [12]	82	PC 12 WON 68	LAMS (AXIOS)	100% 88.2%	1.2%	PCD 5%	Stent mal-deployment 2.5% Bleeding 7.5%
Sharaiha et al. [13]	124	All WON	LAMS (AXIOS)	86.3%	4.8%	10.5%/2.4%	Infection 3.2% Stent occlusion 4% Stent migration 2.4% Bleeding 1.4%
Lakhtakia et al. [14]	205	All WON	Biflanged (Nagi)	96.5%	2.4%	1%/1%	Bleeding 2.9% Perforation 1%
Venkatachalapathy et al. [15]	116	PC 46 WON 70	LAMS (AXIOS)	94%	0.86%	2.5%/–	Sepsis 6% Stent occlusion 0.86% Migration 0.8% Bleeding 0.86% Death 1.7%
Dhir et al. [16]	88	All WON	Biflanged (Nagi)	80.7%	9.1%	Sx 1.1%	Fever 13.6% Stent migration 2.3% Bleeding 3.4%
Yang et al. [17]	122	PC 58 WON 64	LAMS (AXIOS)	96.5% 62.3%	NR	Sx: 3.3% WON	Bleeding 3.3% Infection 4.8%
Kumta et al. [18]	192	PC 41 WON 151	LAMS (AXIOS)	92.6%	3.7%	7.3%/3.1%	Bleeding 5.7% Perforation 2.1% Infection 2.1%
Teoh et al. [19]	59	PC 20 WON 39	LAMS (SPAXUS)	100%	3.4%	None	Bleeding 5.1% Perforation 1.7%

PFC, pancreatic fluid collection; PC, pseudocyst; WON, walled off necrosis; Sx, surgery; PCD, percutaneous drainage; NR, not reported; LAMS, lumen apposing metal stent.

Table 1.
Outcome of endoscopic transmural drainage in pancreatic fluid collections using large caliber metal stents.

several decades now. The proposed advantages of plastic over metal stents include lower cost, less risk of delayed bleeding, and ability to keep them for long term in cases with DPD. On the other hand, metal stents have wider lumen, allowing efficient drainage of the necrotic material and endoscopic necrosectomy when required. Conventional fully covered metal stents used initially were suboptimal due to their longer lengths and lack of lumen apposing properties. The development of novel LCMS has widened the therapeutic armamentarium for ETD of PFCs. Newly developed LCMS have either lumen apposing (AXIOS, Xlumena, Mountain View, CA, United States and Niti-S SPAXUS, TaeWoong Medical Co., Ltd., Ilsan, South Korea) properties or flared ends (NAGI, Taewoong Medical Co, Ilsan, South Korea) to prevent stent migration [10]. As compared to the conventional metal stents, the use of LCMS is associated with superior outcomes in terms of number of procedures required for the resolution of WON [26]. Similarly, better clinical outcomes and reduced requirement of endoscopic necrosectomy have been found with the use of metal stents as compared to plastic stents in several studies [27–30]. In a large, multicenter study including 189 patients with WON, the use of LCMS was associated with higher clinical success (80.4 vs. 57.5%), shorter procedure time, lower need for surgery (5.1 vs. 16.1%), and lower rate of recurrence as compared to plastic stents [31]. However, the superiority of LCMS is not uniform across the published studies. In a randomized trial, there was no significant difference in the treatment outcomes including the total number of procedures performed, treatment success, and readmissions between LCMS and plastic stent groups in patients with WON [24]. In addition, the treatment cost (LCMS: US$12155 vs. plastic stents: US$6609) and stent related adverse events were higher in the LCMS group (32.3 vs. 6.9%, p = 0.01) [24]. Several systematic reviews and meta-analyses draw conflicting conclusions while comparing plastic stents vs. metal stents for ETD of PFCs [32–37]. In three of the published systematic reviews and meta-analyses, metal stents were found superior to plastic stents for both pseudocysts as well as WON in terms of clinical success and adverse events [34, 36, 32]. On the contrary, two other systematic reviews and meta-analyses did not find a difference in the outcomes between metal or plastic stents [33, 37]. It must be emphasized that the paucity of randomized trials is the major limitations of these reviews.

The current trend is to use metal stents for WON with significant debris. These cases may require more frequent re-interventions including endoscopic necrosectomy for which LCMS are ideal. Whereas, plastic stents are an cost effective alternative in pseudocysts or WON with minimal necrotic contents. Randomized trials are warranted before concluding the superiority of metal stents for the management of PFCs.

2.3 Endoscopic necrosectomy

Endoscopic necrosectomy essentially comprises of endoscopic debridement of necrotic debris within the cyst cavity using a variety of methods including DEN and naso-cystic lavage with saline and or diluted hydrogen peroxide (3%, 1:10 dilution). DEN involves the passage of endoscope within the cyst cavity followed by mechanical removal of necrotic tissue using forceps, polypectomy snares, and retrieval nets [38]. With the availability of LCMS (≥15 mm), multiple sessions of DEN can be performed with relative ease. However, there is no dedicated device or accessory for DEN and therefore, the process is cumbersome and time consuming. Recent development of new devices to facilitate endoscopic debridement is likely to make DEN less cumbersome and more efficacious [39, 40].

DEN is safe and effective in about 80–90% of patients with WON. However, DEN may be associated with substantial complications. In a systematic review, the overall rate of adverse events and mortality associated with endoscopic necrosectomy were 22% and 5%, respectively. The complications reported with DEN include air embolism (0.4%), bleeding (11%), and perforation (3%) [41]. Therefore, DEN is usually performed in cases with no improvement after ETD alone.

Our group re-defined the endoscopic step-up approach in patients with WON. This approach includes cyst cavity lavage using nasocystic catheter and de-clogging of the metal stent as intermediate steps after transmural placement of metal stent and before proceeding to endoscopic necrosectomy [14]. With this approach, endoscopic necrosectomy can be avoided in the vast majority of patients with WON.

2.4 Step-up approach for walled of necrosis

Open surgery is associated with a high morbidity and mortality in patients with WON. Consequently, minimally invasive surgical or endoscopic approaches have virtually replaced open necrosectomy in these patients [6]. The available evidence favors a step-up approach over the conventional techniques [7, 42–44]. In general, minimally invasive surgical step-up approach consists of percutaneous drainage followed by (if necessary) video assisted retroperitoneal debridement (VARD). Whereas, endoscopic step up approach includes ETD followed by (if necessary) endoscopic necrosectomy. Percutaneous catheter drainage can be used as an adjunct to ETD in cases with incomplete response or large collections with extension into paracolic gutter (**Figure 6**).

Several trials have compared endoscopic versus minimally invasive surgical methods of drainage in cases with WON [7, 45]. In a randomized trial by the Dutch Pancreatitis Study Group, there was no difference in the incidence of major complications or mortality between the endoscopic or minimally invasive surgical step-up approach (endoscopy: 43% vs. surgery: 45%, p = 0.88) [7]. However, the rate of

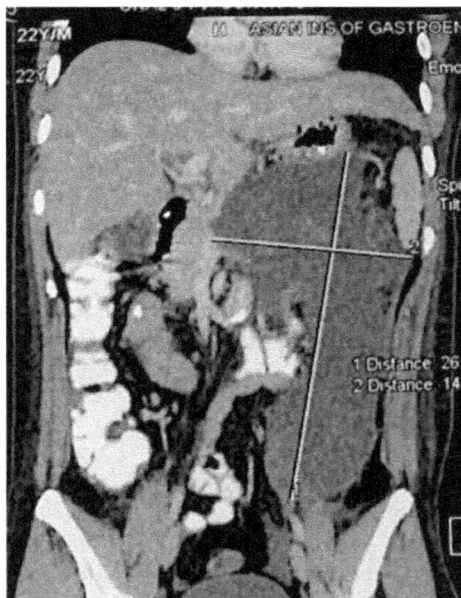

Figure 6.
Large pancreatic fluid collection extending into pelvis.

pancreatic fistulas (5 vs 32%, p < 0.01) and the length of hospital stay were lower in the endoscopy group [7]. In another randomized trial including 66 patients with infected WON, ETD was associated with significantly reduced major complications (0.15 vs. 0.69), lowered costs (75,830 $ vs. 117,492 $), lower incidence of pancreatic fistula (0 vs. 28.1%), and increased quality of life as compared to minimally invasive surgery [45]. In a recent systematic review including two randomized trials and four observational studies, ETD was associated with lower mortality, risk of major organ failure, adverse events, and length of hospital stay [44]. These trials suggest that endoscopic step-up approach should be preferred over minimally invasive surgical step-up approach for the management of PFCs.

2.5 Endoscopic vs. surgical drainage: pseudocysts

Endoscopic and surgical cyst-gastrostomy have been compared in several studies [46–50]. Initial non-randomized trials found surgical drainage to be superior to endoscopic drainage of pseudocysts [50]. However, subsequent randomized studies concluded that endoscopic drainage achieves similar outcomes as compared to surgical drainage [46, 49, 47]. In addition, EUS guided cyst-gastrostomy is less invasive, cost saving, and associated with a shorter length of a post procedure hospital stay when compared with surgical cyst-gastrostomy [46, 47]. In a recent systematic review and meta-analysis including six studies (342 patients), there was no significant difference between surgical and endoscopic treatment success rates, adverse events, and recurrence for pancreatic pseudocysts [51]. To conclude, the current evidence suggests that endoscopic drainage is as efficacious as surgical cyst-gastrostomy for pseudocysts with shorter hospital stay and reduced costs.

2.6 Endoscopic vs. percutaneous drainage

Percutaneous catheter drainage remains an important modality even in the era of minimally invasive endoscopic or surgical treatments. In different studies, percutaneous drainage alone was successful in 35–50% of cases with WON [52]. Percutaneous drainage can be used as an adjunctive to endoscopic drainage in selected cases with large PFCs extending into paracolic gutters or pelvis. In addition, percutaneous drainage is useful in acute or ill-defined PFCs (<4 weeks) where endoscopic drainage may not be feasible. Percutaneous tract can also be utilized for endoscopic and VARD [43]. Having described all the major advantages of percutaneous catheter drainage, the major limitation remains the development of external pancreatocutaneous fistula which may be difficult to treat.

As compared to percutaneous approach, endoscopic drainage is associated with significantly better clinical success, a lower re-intervention rate, and a shorter hospital length of stay [53]. Therefore, percutaneous drainage is only performed in cases where either endoscopic drainage is not available or not feasible (ill-defined or distantly located collections).

2.7 Dual modality drainage

Dual modality drainage (DMD) involves the simultaneous or sequential use of endoscopic and percutaneous approaches for symptomatic PFCs. Several studies have concluded the utility of DMD in symptomatic PFCs especially WON [54, 55]. The proposed advantages of this technique include a quicker recovery and reduced chances of forming an external pancreato-cutaneous fistula. In the study by Gluck et al., the use of DMD was associated with reduced length of hospital stay, and less requirement of radiological or endoscopic interventions [55].

This technique may be especially useful in cases with large WON especially those extending into the paracolic gutters [56]. In these cases, transmural approach alone may not provide adequate drainage in these patients (**Figure 6**).

2.8 Trans-papillary drainage of PFCs

Trans-papillary drainage (TPD) of PFCs may be useful in certain scenarios as follows: (a) small size of cyst (<5 cm) communicating with main pancreatic duct (PD), (b) as an adjunct to ETD in cases with PD leak or disconnected PD, (c) chronic pancreatitis with an obstructed PD communicating with a pseudocyst, and (d) management of external pancreatic fistula after percutaneous or surgical drainage [22]. When used as a primary modality, TPD provides the path of least resistance for the pancreatic juice, thereby diverting it away from the cyst. There is a potential of cyst infection with TPD and therefore, antibiotics should be routinely given to these patients. TPD may be useful in preventing recurrences of PFCs following ETD in cases with PD leak and disconnected PD [57]. We do not routinely perform TPD as an adjunct to ETD in all the cases. In our practice, we evaluate the PD anatomy using an magnetic resonance cholangio-pancreatogram (MRCP) prior to removal of stents placed during ETD. In cases with a PD stricture, leak or disconnection we attempt placing a trans-papillary PD stent. Subsequently, trans-papillary stents are removed or exchanged (as per the PD morphology) after 4–6 weeks. However, trans-papillary stenting may not be always feasible especially in cases with a disconnected PD. In these cases, transmural plastic stents can be left in situ and metal stents can be exchanged with plastic stents [58]. However, the latter approach needs to be substantiated by high quality randomized studies. Nevertheless, metal stents should be removed between 2 and 4 weeks irrespective of the PD anatomy due to the risk of buried stent syndrome and delayed bleeding.

2.9 Endoscopic drainage of PFC in children

The literature regarding the efficacy of endoscopic drainage of PFCs in children is sparse. Unlike adults, the feasibility of drainage using an adult duodenoscope or EUS scope is questionable in smaller children. Nevertheless, emerging data indicates that EUS-guided drainage is feasible and effective in children with PFCs [59–63]. Our group evaluated the long-term outcomes in 30 children with PFCs using pigtail plastic stents [60]. Clinical success was documented in 93% of children at a median follow up of 829 days. The use of novel metal stents has also been described in pediatric age group [62, 61]. Nabi et al. used novel bi-flanged metal stents in 21 children with WON. Metal stents could be successfully placed in all the children, and clinical success was achieved in 95% of children [62].

3. Recent advancements

The technique of ETD of PFCs using metal stents requires a series of steps including needle puncture, coiling of guidewire in the cyst cavity, balloon dilatation of the cystogastric tract, and finally, deployment of stent. With the availability of electrocautery-enhanced delivery systems, the deployment of metal stents can be achieved in a single step [64, 65]. Therefore, the drainage of PFCs using these "Hot Devices" is quicker and simpler. Currently, the electrocautery-enhanced delivery system is available with lumen apposing (Hot *AXIOS*) as well as biflanged metal stents (Hot *NAGI*).

4. Individualized approach to pancreatic fluid collections

The management of PFCs requires an individualized approach based on their maturity (acute or well defined), contents, and anatomical location in relation to gastroduodenal wall (**Figure 7**). Asymptomatic PFCs do not require drainage irrespective of their size. Similarly, symptomatic and ill-defined APFCs are managed conservatively with antibiotics (if necessary), nutritional support, and analgesics initially. In non-responders, percutaneous drainage is a reasonable next step in acute collections.

Mature PFCs with a well-defined wall and in close proximity to gastroduodenal wall can be managed endoscopically using plastic or metal endoprostheses in majority of the cases. We prefer LCMS in PFCs containing substantial necrotic debris identified on EUS or MRI. Occasionally, the PFC is situated away (>1–1.5 cm) from the gastroduodenal wall and not amenable to endoscopic drainage. In these cases, percutaneous or minimally invasive surgical drainage (e.g., VARD) are alternatives.

Subsequent interventions are carried in a step-up fashion based on the persistence of significant symptoms. Endoscopic or percutaneous necrosectomy is performed in non-responders who underwent ETD or percutaneous drainage, respectively, as the primary mode of drainage. We prefer intermediary steps including naso-cystic lavage and de-clogging of LCMS before proceeding to DEN. In our experience, only a minor fraction of cases require DEN with this approach [14]. Some cases do not respond to the aforementioned minimally invasive step-up approach and require an open surgical debridement.

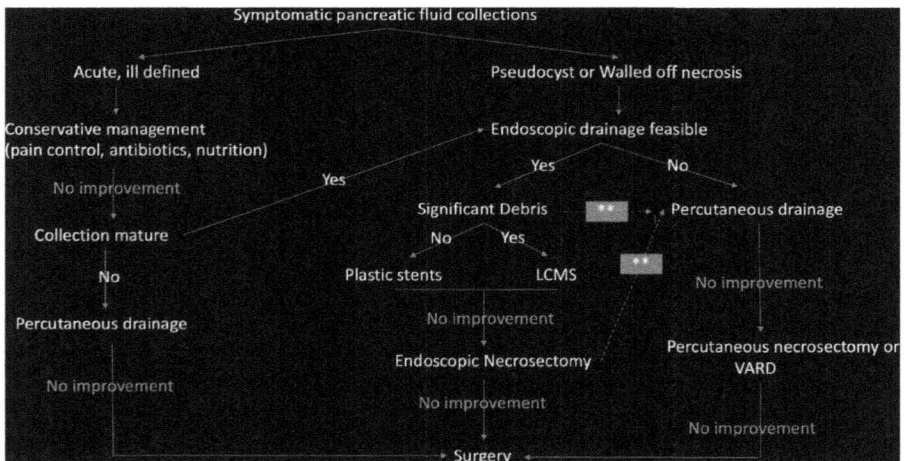

Figure 7.
*Approach to symptomatic pancreatic fluid collections. VARD, video-assisted retroperitoneal debridement; LCMS, large caliber metal stent; **percutaneous drainage can be performed either simultaneously with endoscopic transmural drainage or sequentially in non-responders.*

5. Conclusions

The management of PFCs requires a multidisciplinary approach involving experienced endoscopists, interventional radiologists, pancreatic surgeons, and nutritionists. Endoscopic drainage is the preferred first line approach to symptomatic and infected PFCs. Percutaneous drainage is useful in selected scenarios and can complement the benefits of endotherapy in large collections extending toward pelvis. The approach to PFCs should not be rigid and should be individualized for each patient. In general, a step-up approach minimizes the morbidity associated with open surgical drainage and is usually successful in majority of the patients. However, some cases do require open surgical debridement despite of all the recent advancements in endotherapy.

Author details

Zaheer Nabi* and D. Nageshwar Reddy
Asian Institute of Gastroenterology, Hyderabad, India

*Address all correspondence to: zaheernabi1978@gmail.com

IntechOpen

References

[1] Banks PA, Bollen TL, Dervenis C, Gooszen HG, Johnson CD, Sarr MG, et al. Classification of acute pancreatitis–2012: Revision of the Atlanta classification and definitions by international consensus. Gut. 2013;**62**(1):102-111. DOI: 10.1136/gutjnl-2012-302779

[2] Manrai M, Kochhar R, Gupta V, Yadav TD, Dhaka N, Kalra N, et al. Outcome of acute pancreatic and peripancreatic collections occurring in patients with acute pancreatitis. Annals of Surgery. 2018;**267**(2):357-363. DOI: 10.1097/SLA.0000000000002065

[3] Sarathi Patra P, Das K, Bhattacharyya A, Ray S, Hembram J, Sanyal S, et al. Natural resolution or intervention for fluid collections in acute severe pancreatitis. The British Journal of Surgery. 2014;**101**(13):1721-1728. DOI: 10.1002/bjs.9666

[4] Cui ML, Kim KH, Kim HG, Han J, Kim H, Cho KB, et al. Incidence, risk factors and clinical course of pancreatic fluid collections in acute pancreatitis. Digestive Diseases and Sciences. 2014;**59**(5):1055-1062. DOI: 10.1007/s10620-013-2967-4

[5] van Santvoort HC, Besselink MG, Bakker OJ, Hofker HS, Boermeester MA, Dejong CH, et al. A step-up approach or open necrosectomy for necrotizing pancreatitis. The New England Journal of Medicine. 2010;**362**(16):1491-1502. DOI: 10.1056/NEJMoa0908821

[6] van Brunschot S, Hollemans RA, Bakker OJ, Besselink MG, Baron TH, Beger HG, et al. Minimally invasive and endoscopic versus open necrosectomy for necrotising pancreatitis: A pooled analysis of individual data for 1980 patients. Gut. 2018;**67**(4):697-706. DOI: 10.1136/gutjnl-2016-313341

[7] van Brunschot S, van Grinsven J, van Santvoort HC, Bakker OJ, Besselink MG, Boermeester MA, et al. Endoscopic or surgical step-up approach for infected necrotising pancreatitis: A multicentre randomised trial. Lancet. 2018;**391**(10115):51-58. DOI: 10.1016/S0140-6736(17)32404-2

[8] Bausch D, Wellner U, Kahl S, Kuesters S, Richter-Schrag HJ, Utzolino S, et al. Minimally invasive operations for acute necrotizing pancreatitis: Comparison of minimally invasive retroperitoneal necrosectomy with endoscopic transgastric necrosectomy. Surgery. 2012;**152** (3 Suppl 1):S128-S134. DOI: 10.1016/j.surg.2012.05.021

[9] Bakker OJ, van Santvoort HC, van Brunschot S, Geskus RB, Besselink MG, Bollen TL, et al. Endoscopic transgastric vs surgical necrosectomy for infected necrotizing pancreatitis: A randomized trial. Journal of the American Medical Association. 2012;**307**(10):1053-1061. DOI: 10.1001/jama.2012.276

[10] Nabi Z, Basha J, Reddy DN. Endoscopic management of pancreatic fluid collections-revisited. World Journal of Gastroenterology. 2017;**23**(15):2660-2672. DOI: 10.3748/wjg.v23.i15.2660

[11] Walter D, Will U, Sanchez-Yague A, Brenke D, Hampe J, Wollny H, et al. A novel lumen-apposing metal stent for endoscopic ultrasound-guided drainage of pancreatic fluid collections: A prospective cohort study. Endoscopy. 2015;**47**(1):63-67. DOI: 10.1055/s-0034-1378113

[12] Siddiqui AA, Adler DG, Nieto J, Shah JN, Binmoeller KF, Kane S, et al. EUS-guided drainage of peripancreatic fluid collections and necrosis by using a novel lumen-apposing stent: A large retrospective, multicenter U.S. experience (with videos). Gastrointestinal Endoscopy.

2016;**83**(4):699-707. DOI: 10.1016/j.
gie.2015.10.020

[13] Sharaiha RZ, Tyberg A,
Khashab MA, Kumta NA, Karia K,
Nieto J, et al. Endoscopic therapy with
lumen-apposing metal stents is
safe and effective for patients with
pancreatic walled-off necrosis. Clinical
Gastroenterology and Hepatology.
2016;**14**(12):1797-1803. DOI: 10.1016/j.
cgh.2016.05.011

[14] Lakhtakia S, Basha J, Talukdar R,
Gupta R, Nabi Z, Ramchandani M, et al.
Endoscopic "step-up approach" using a
dedicated biflanged metal stent reduces
the need for direct necrosectomy in
walled-off necrosis (with videos).
Gastrointestinal Endoscopy.
2017;**85**(6):1243-1252. DOI: 10.1016/j.
gie.2016.10.037

[15] Venkatachalapathy SV, Bekkali N,
Pereira S, Johnson G, Oppong K,
Nayar M, et al. Multicenter experience
from the UK and Ireland of
use of lumen-apposing metal
stent for transluminal drainage
of pancreatic fluid collections.
Endoscopy International Open.
2018;**6**(3):E259-EE65. DOI:
10.1055/s-0043-125362

[16] Dhir V, Adler DG, Dalal A,
Aherrao N, Shah R, Maydeo A. Early
removal of biflanged metal stents in
the management of pancreatic walled-
off necrosis: A prospective study.
Endoscopy. 2018;**50**(6):597-605. DOI:
10.1055/s-0043-123575

[17] Yang D, Perbtani YB, Mramba LK,
Kerdsirichairat T, Prabhu A, Manvar A,
et al. Safety and rate of delayed adverse
events with lumen-apposing metal
stents (LAMS) for pancreatic fluid
collections: A multicenter study.
Endoscopy International Open.
2018;**6**(10):E1267-E1E75. DOI:
10.1055/a-0732-502

[18] Kumta NA, Tyberg A, Bhagat VH,
Siddiqui AA, Kowalski TE, Loren DE,

et al. EUS-guided drainage of pancreatic
fluid collections using lumen apposing
metal stents: An international,
multicenter experience. Digestive and
Liver Disease. 2019. DOI: 10.1016/j.
dld.2019.05.033

[19] Teoh AYB, Bapaye A, Lakhtakia S,
Ratanachu T, Reknimitr R, Chan SM,
et al. Prospective multicenter
international study on the outcomes of
a newly developed self-approximating
lumen-apposing metallic stent for
drainage of pancreatic fluid collections
and endoscopic necrosectomy. Digestive
Endoscopy. 2019. DOI: 10.1111/
den.13494

[20] Guo J, Duan B, Sun S, Wang S,
Liu X, Ge N, et al. Multivariate analysis
of the factors affecting the prognosis
of walled-off pancreatic necrosis after
endoscopic ultrasound-guided drainage.
Surgical Endoscopy. 2019. DOI: 10.1007/
s00464-019-06870-3

[21] Bang JY, Wilcox CM,
Navaneethan U, Hasan MK, Peter S,
Christein J, et al. Impact of disconnected
pancreatic duct syndrome on the
endoscopic management of pancreatic
fluid collections. Annals of Surgery.
2018;**267**(3):561-568. DOI: 10.1097/
SLA.0000000000002082

[22] Elmunzer BJ. Endoscopic drainage
of pancreatic fluid collections. Clinical
Gastroenterology and Hepatology.
2018;**16**(12):1851-1863. DOI: 10.1016/j.
cgh.2018.03.021

[23] Lang GD, Fritz C, Bhat T, Das KK,
Murad FM, Early DS, et al. EUS-guided
drainage of peripancreatic fluid
collections with lumen-apposing metal
stents and plastic double-pigtail stents:
Comparison of efficacy and adverse
event rates. Gastrointestinal Endoscopy.
2018;**87**(1):150-157. DOI: 10.1016/j.
gie.2017.06.029

[24] Bang JY, Navaneethan U, Hasan MK,
Sutton B, Hawes R, Varadarajulu S. Non-

superiority of lumen-apposing metal stents over plastic stents for drainage of walled-off necrosis in a randomised trial. Gut. 2019;**68**(7):1200-1209. DOI: 10.1136/gutjnl-2017-315335

[25] Brimhall B, Han S, Tatman PD, Clark TJ, Wani S, Brauer B, et al. Increased incidence of pseudoaneurysm bleeding with lumen-apposing metal stents compared to double-pigtail plastic stents in patients with peripancreatic fluid collections. Clinical Gastroenterology and Hepatology. 2018;**16**(9):1521-1528. DOI: 10.1016/j.cgh.2018.02.021

[26] Siddiqui AA, Kowalski TE, Loren DE, Khalid A, Soomro A, Mazhar SM, et al. Fully covered self-expanding metal stents versus lumen-apposing fully covered self-expanding metal stent versus plastic stents for endoscopic drainage of pancreatic walled-off necrosis: Clinical outcomes and success. Gastrointestinal Endoscopy. 2017;**85**(4):758-765. DOI: 10.1016/j.gie.2016.08.014

[27] Abu Dayyeh BK, Mukewar S, Majumder S, Zaghlol R, Vargas Valls EJ, Bazerbachi F, et al. Large-caliber metal stents versus plastic stents for the management of pancreatic walled-off necrosis. Gastrointestinal Endoscopy. 2018;**87**(1):141-149. DOI: 10.1016/j.gie.2017.04.032

[28] Bapaye A, Dubale NA, Sheth KA, Bapaye J, Ramesh J, Gadhikar H, et al. Endoscopic ultrasonography-guided transmural drainage of walled-off pancreatic necrosis: Comparison between a specially designed fully covered bi-flanged metal stent and multiple plastic stents. Digestive Endoscopy. 2017;**29**(1):104-110. DOI: 10.1111/den.12704

[29] Chen YI, Barkun AN, Adam V, Bai G, Singh VK, Bukhari M, et al. Cost-effectiveness analysis comparing lumen-apposing metal stents with plastic

stents in the management of pancreatic walled-off necrosis. Gastrointestinal Endoscopy. 2018;**88**(2):267-276. DOI: 10.1016/j.gie.2018.03.021

[30] Sharaiha RZ, DeFilippis EM, Kedia P, Gaidhane M, Boumitri C, Lim HW, et al. Metal versus plastic for pancreatic pseudocyst drainage: Clinical outcomes and success. Gastrointestinal Endoscopy. 2015;**82**(5):822-827. DOI: 10.1016/j.gie.2015.02.035

[31] Chen YI, Yang J,Friedland S, Holmes I, Law R, Hosmer A, et al. Lumen apposing metal stents are superior to plastic stents in pancreatic walled-off necrosis: A large international multicenter study. Endoscopy International Open. 2019;7(3):E347-EE54. DOI: 10.1055/a-0828-7630

[32] Bazerbachi F, Sawas T, Vargas EJ, Prokop LJ, Chari ST, Gleeson FC, et al. Metal stents versus plastic stents for the management of pancreatic walled-off necrosis: A systematic review and meta-analysis. Gastrointestinal Endoscopy. 2018;**87**(1):30-42. DOI: 10.1016/j.gie.2017.08.025

[33] Mohan BP, Jayaraj M, Asokkumar R, Shakhatreh M, Pahal P, Ponnada S, et al. Lumen apposing metal stents in drainage of pancreatic walled-off necrosis, are they any better than plastic stents? A systematic review and meta-analysis of studies published since the revised Atlanta classification of pancreatic fluid collections. Endoscopic ultrasound. 2019;**8**(2):82-90. DOI: 10.4103/eus.eus_7_19

[34] Hammad T, Khan MA, Alastal Y, Lee W, Nawras A, Ismail MK, et al. Efficacy and safety of lumen-apposing metal stents in management of pancreatic fluid collections: Are they better than plastic stents? A systematic review and meta-analysis. Digestive Diseases and Sciences. 2018;**63**(2):289-301. DOI: 10.1007/s10620-017-4851-0

[35] Renelus BD, Jamorabo DS, Gurm HK, Dave N, Briggs WM, Arya M. Comparative outcomes of endoscopic ultrasound-guided cystogastrostomy for peripancreatic fluid collections: A systematic review and meta-analysis. Therapeutic Advances in Gastrointestinal Endoscopy. 2019;**12**:2631774519843400. DOI: 10.1177/2631774519843400

[36] Yoon SB, Lee IS, Choi MG. Metal versus plastic stents for drainage of pancreatic fluid collection: A meta-analysis. United European Gastroenterology Journal. 2018;**6**(5):729-738. DOI: 10.1177/2050640618761702

[37] Bang JY, Hawes R, Bartolucci A, Varadarajulu S. Efficacy of metal and plastic stents for transmural drainage of pancreatic fluid collections: A systematic review. Digestive Endoscopy. 2015;**27**(4):486-498. DOI: 10.1111/den.12418

[38] Baron TH, DiMaio CJ, Wang AY, Morgan KA. American Gastroenterological Association clinical practice update: Management of pancreatic necrosis. Gastroenterology. 2019. DOI: 10.1053/j.gastro.2019.07.064

[39] Wiel SE, Poley JW, Grubben M, Bruno MJ, Koch AD. The EndoRotor, a novel tool for the endoscopic management of pancreatic necrosis. Endoscopy. 2018;**50**(9):E240-E2E1. DOI: 10.1055/a-0628-6136

[40] Bazarbashi AN, Ge PS, de Moura DTH, Thompson CC. A novel endoscopic morcellator device to facilitate direct necrosectomy of solid walled-off necrosis. Endoscopy. 2019. DOI: 10.1055/a-0956-6605

[41] Luigiano C, Pellicano R, Fusaroli P, Iabichino G, Arena M, Lisotti A, et al. Pancreatic necrosectomy: An evidence-based systematic review of the levels of evidence and a comparison of endoscopic versus non-endoscopic techniques. Minerva Chirurgica. 2016;**71**(4):262-269

[42] Nemoto Y, Attam R, Arain MA, Trikudanathan G, Mallery S, Beilman GJ, et al. Interventions for walled off necrosis using an algorithm based endoscopic step-up approach: Outcomes in a large cohort of patients. Pancreatology. 2017;**17**(5):663-668. DOI: 10.1016/j.pan.2017.07.195

[43] Jain S, Padhan R, Bopanna S, Jain SK, Dhingra R, Dash NR, et al. Percutaneous endoscopic step-up therapy is an effective minimally invasive approach for infected necrotizing pancreatitis. Digestive Diseases and Sciences. 2019. DOI: 10.1007/s10620-019-05696-2

[44] Khan MA, Kahaleh M, Khan Z, Tyberg A, Solanki S, Haq KF, et al. Time for a changing of guard: From minimally invasive surgery to endoscopic drainage for management of pancreatic walled-off necrosis. Journal of Clinical Gastroenterology. 2019;**53**(2):81-88. DOI: 10.1097/MCG.0000000000001141

[45] Bang JY, Arnoletti JP, Holt BA, Sutton B, Hasan MK, Navaneethan U, et al. An endoscopic transluminal approach, compared with minimally invasive surgery, reduces complications and costs for patients with necrotizing pancreatitis. Gastroenterology. 2019;**156**(4):1027-1040. DOI: 10.1053/j.gastro.2018.11.031

[46] Varadarajulu S, Lopes TL, Wilcox CM, Drelichman ER, Kilgore ML, Christein JD. EUS versus surgical cyst-gastrostomy for management of pancreatic pseudocysts. Gastrointestinal Endoscopy. 2008;**68**(4):649-655. DOI: 10.1016/j.gie.2008.02.057

[47] Varadarajulu S, Bang JY, Sutton BS, Trevino JM, Christein JD, Wilcox CM. Equal efficacy

of endoscopic and surgical cystogastrostomy for pancreatic pseudocyst drainage in a randomized trial. Gastroenterology. 2013;**145**(3):583-590. DOI: 10.1053/j.gastro.2013.05.046

[48] Saul A, Ramirez Luna MA, Chan C, Uscanga L, Valdovinos Andraca F, Hernandez Calleros J, et al. EUS-guided drainage of pancreatic pseudocysts offers similar success and complications compared to surgical treatment but with a lower cost. Surgical Endoscopy. 2016;**30**(4):1459-1465. DOI: 10.1007/s00464-015-4351-2

[49] Garg PK, Meena D, Babu D, Padhan RK, Dhingra R, Krishna A, et al. Endoscopic versus laparoscopic drainage of pseudocyst and walled-off necrosis following acute pancreatitis: A randomized trial. Surgical Endoscopy. 2019. DOI: 10.1007/s00464-019-06866-z

[50] Melman L, Azar R, Beddow K, Brunt LM, Halpin VJ, Eagon JC, et al. Primary and overall success rates for clinical outcomes after laparoscopic, endoscopic, and open pancreatic cystgastrostomy for pancreatic pseudocysts. Surgical Endoscopy. 2009;**23**(2):267-271. DOI: 10.1007/s00464-008-0196-2

[51] Farias GFA, Bernardo WM, De Moura DTH, Guedes HG, Brunaldi VO, Visconti TAC, et al. Endoscopic versus surgical treatment for pancreatic pseudocysts: Systematic review and meta-analysis. Medicine (Baltimore). 2019;**98**(8):e14255. DOI: 10.1097/MD.0000000000014255

[52] van Baal MC, van Santvoort HC, Bollen TL, Bakker OJ, Besselink MG, Gooszen HG, et al. Systematic review of percutaneous catheter drainage as primary treatment for necrotizing pancreatitis. The British Journal of Surgery. 2011;**98**(1):18-27. DOI: 10.1002/bjs.7304

[53] Khan MA, Hammad T, Khan Z, Lee W, Gaidhane M, Tyberg A, et al.

Endoscopic versus percutaneous management for symptomatic pancreatic fluid collections: A systematic review and meta-analysis. Endoscopy International Open. 2018;**6**(4):E474-EE83. DOI: 10.1055/s-0044-102299

[54] Ross AS, Irani S, Gan SI, Rocha F, Siegal J, Fotoohi M, et al. Dual-modality drainage of infected and symptomatic walled-off pancreatic necrosis: Long-term clinical outcomes. Gastrointestinal Endoscopy. 2014;**79**(6):929-935. DOI: 10.1016/j.gie.2013.10.014

[55] Gluck M, Ross A, Irani S, Lin O, Gan SI, Fotoohi M, et al. Dual modality drainage for symptomatic walled-off pancreatic necrosis reduces length of hospitalization, radiological procedures, and number of endoscopies compared to standard percutaneous drainage. Journal of Gastrointestinal Surgery. 2012;**16**(2):248-256. DOI: 10.1007/s11605-011-1759-4

[56] Papachristou GI, Takahashi N, Chahal P, Sarr MG, Baron TH. Peroral endoscopic drainage/debridement of walled-off pancreatic necrosis. Annals of Surgery. 2007;**245**(6):943-951. DOI: 10.1097/01.sla.0000254366.19366.69

[57] Arvanitakis M, Delhaye M, Bali MA, Matos C, De Maertelaer V, Le Moine O, et al. Pancreatic-fluid collections: A randomized controlled trial regarding stent removal after endoscopic transmural drainage. Gastrointestinal Endoscopy. 2007;**65**(4):609-619. DOI: 10.1016/j.gie.2006.06.083

[58] Varadarajulu S, Wilcox CM. Endoscopic placement of permanent indwelling transmural stents in disconnected pancreatic duct syndrome: Does benefit outweigh the risks? Gastrointestinal Endoscopy. 2011;**74**(6):1408-1412. DOI: 10.1016/j.gie.2011.07.049

[59] Bang JY, Varadarajulu S. Endoscopic treatment of walled-off necrosis

in children: Clinical experience and treatment outcomes. Journal of Pediatric Gastroenterology and Nutrition. 2016;**63**(3):e31-e35. DOI: 10.1097/MPG.0000000000001269

[60] Nabi Z, Lakhtakia S, Basha J, Chavan R, Gupta R, Ramchandani M, et al. Endoscopic drainage of pancreatic fluid collections: Long-term outcomes in children. Digestive Endoscopy. 2017;**29**(7):790-797. DOI: 10.1111/den.12884

[61] Giefer MJ, Balmadrid BL. Pediatric application of the lumen-apposing metal stent for pancreatic fluid collections. Gastrointestinal Endoscopy. 2016;**84**(1):188-189. DOI: 10.1016/j.gie.2016.01.045

[62] Nabi Z, Lakhtakia S, Basha J, Chavan R, Ramchandani M, Gupta R, et al. Endoscopic ultrasound-guided drainage of walled-off necrosis in children with fully covered self-expanding metal stents. Journal of Pediatric Gastroenterology and Nutrition. 2017;**64**(4):592-597. DOI: 10.1097/MPG.0000000000001491

[63] Ramesh J, Bang JY, Trevino J, Varadarajulu S. Endoscopic ultrasound-guided drainage of pancreatic fluid collections in children. Journal of Pediatric Gastroenterology and Nutrition. 2013;**56**(1):30-35. DOI: 10.1097/MPG.0b013e318267c113

[64] Lakhtakia S, Nabi Z, Moon JH, Gupta R, Chavan R, Basha J, et al. Endoscopic drainage of pancreatic fluid collections by use of a novel biflanged stent with electrocautery-enhanced delivery system. VideoGIE. 2018;**3**(9):284-288. DOI: 10.1016/j.vgie.2018.07.001

[65] Rinninella E, Kunda R, Dollhopf M, Sanchez-Yague A, Will U, Tarantino I, et al. EUS-guided drainage of pancreatic fluid collections using a novel lumen-apposing metal stent on an electrocautery-enhanced delivery system: A large retrospective study (with video). Gastrointestinal Endoscopy. 2015;**82**(6):1039-1046. DOI: 10.1016/j.gie.2015.04.006

Chapter 3

Endoscopic Management of Pancreatic Fluid Collection in Acute Pancreatitis

Cosmas Rinaldi Adithya Lesmana,
Laurentius Adrianto Lesmana and Khek Yu Ho

Abstract

Acute pancreatitis is an acute clinical condition where it can be manifested as mild disease or serious and life-threatening condition. There are several factors that may be responsible for this condition, such as genetic, gallstone disease, alcohol consumption, pancreatic trauma, medication, hypertriglyceridemia, autoimmune disease, and surgery. The most common manifestation of pancreatic parenchymal injury is pancreatic pseudocyst (PPC) formation, where peripancreatic fluid collection (PFCs) usually precedes this condition. Even though most of the pseudocyst can be managed conservatively, however in conditions such as infected pseudocyst or possible wall of necrosis (WON), there should be an early intervention management. Clinical evaluation and imaging studies have to be done in the beginning. Computed tomography (CT) scan or magnetic resonance imaging (MRI) are the main imaging techniques used to evaluate the characteristic of the cyst, the size, surrounding vascularity, and to assess the pancreatic duct itself with possible of fistula formation. Clinical conditions that are usually considered for early intervention management are symptomatic pseudocyst, large size of pseudocyst, presence of gastric outlet obstruction, or biliary obstruction. PFC should be evaluated as it has been classified based on type of pancreatitis, time frame, well-defined wall, and debris contained inside the cyst. Endoscopic management has replaced percutaneous and surgical approach in most of PFC cases. Nowadays, endoscopic ultrasound (EUS) has been widely used as the first-line tool for PFC drainage procedure. Pancreatic pseudocyst stenting is the most common procedure in most of the centers in the world. However, the cost, availability, and expertise are needed to be considered in clinical practice.

Keywords: endoscopic management, pancreatic fluid collections, acute pancreatitis

1. Introduction

Acute pancreatitis is one of the challenging situations in clinical practice where it can lead to a critical condition. This condition also needs to be carefully managed to prevent more complications [1]. One of the major complications is acute peripancreatic fluid collections (APPFC) and pseudocyst development [2, 3]. The clinical

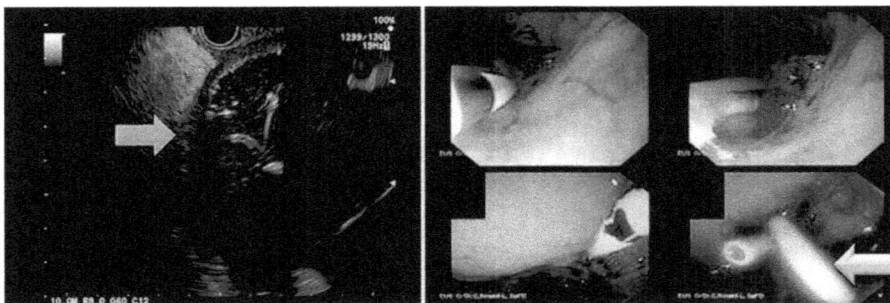

Figure 1.
Patient with infected pancreatic pseudocyst and acute pancreatitis [6].

decision for pancreatic pseudocyst or necrotic infected cyst drainage procedure is very important with regard to the patient's clinical condition and imaging evaluation. There are several well-known routes of drainage procedure of choice such as percutaneous, endoscopic, or surgical drainage [4].

Recently, development of therapeutic endoscopic ultrasound (EUS) procedure has become more popular in most of the highly experienced centers as a first-line management in pancreatic fluid collection drainage [5–7] (**Figure 1**). However, it would need a good comprehensive team work and facilities to perform this kind of procedure.

2. Acute pancreatitis and pancreatic fluid collection

Acute pancreatitis is an acute clinical condition due to sudden inflammation of the pancreas, and it is mostly caused by gallstone disease or alcohol consumption. The other risks of acute pancreatitis are endoscopic retrograde cholangiopancreatography (ERCP) procedure, some medications, trauma of the abdomen, autoimmune disease, hypertriglyceridemia, hereditary factors, abnormalities of the pancreas anatomy, infection, surgical procedure, and pancreatic tumor. Acute pancreatitis consists of two phases of disease: (1) within 1 week, where the systemic inflammation plays an important role and it can be accompanied by organ failure; and (2) more than 1 week, where local complications happened, such as acute peripancreatic fluid collections (APPFC), acute necrotic fluid collection (ANC), pancreatic pseudocyst (PPC), and walled-off necrosis (WON), either can be sterile or infected. This has been classified based on the revised Atlanta criteria. This criteria has been mainly based on time after the onset (whether it is ≤4 weeks or >4 weeks from the onset of pain) and whether there is a necrosis condition through the imaging examination [7, 8]. Acute pancreatitis can be easily diagnosed based on three classic parameters, which are abdominal pain, serum amylase, and/or lipase more than three times upper limit normal, and abdominal imaging study. Abdominal ultrasound should be routinely performed in acute pancreatitis patients as gallstone disease is still the most common etiology. This issue is important to consider early cholecystectomy to prevent more complications in the pancreas [9].

On the other hand, the development of PFC can also be subdivided into early complication (APPFC and ANC) and delayed complication (PPC and WON). APPFC, which contains sterile pancreatic juice, is usually developed within 48 h in almost 50% acute pancreatitis patients, where this condition might be resolved within 2–4 weeks. In the imaging study, homogeneous fluid attenuation conforms to the retroperitoneal structures without any wall which is the hallmark.

Meanwhile, ANC can be located pancreatic, peripancreatic, or mixed. It is usually arising from the necrotic pancreas tissue or glandular and mostly it is connected to the pancreatic duct. Imaging study showed inhomogeneous without any liquefied components and wall. If the fluid collection persists, then usually it can further lead to the development of PPC. PPC is a pancreatic juice collection surrounded by the wall. The location of pseudocyst development usually is at the lesser sac. The cyst wall is formed from the fibrous or granulomatous tissue. Based on imaging studies, it is an oval-round cystic lesion with a thin-walled even though sometimes the wall can be thicker. More than 50% of PPC are usually either resolved or drained spontaneously into the stomach. The larger size of PPC can cause symptoms such as abdominal pain or rupture into the peritoneal cavity. Other related complications are secondary infection, internal bleeding, and bile duct or duodenal obstruction. WON is the transformation of pseudocyst and ANC; it is a thick cavity wall containing semi-liquid collection and necrotic debris. Based on the imaging study, there is an inhomogeneous nonliquefied component encapsulated with wall. Imaging studies are very important to differentiate each of PFC types, as it will have different management and prognosis [10, 11].

3. Endoscopic management of pancreatic fluid collection: history and development

Traditionally, percutaneous and surgical approaches are the old standard methods for PFC (PPC and WON) drainage, where the percutaneous approach can be performed easily for PPC drainage with transabdominal ultrasound-guided or computed tomography (CT) guide. Meanwhile, the surgical approach is the usually preferred method, especially for ANC or WON. It is an open approach and consists of cystogastrostomy, cystoduodenostomy, and cystojejunostomy. Laparoscopic method for PFC drainage was also increasingly reported afterward. However, looking at the high complication rate of surgery approach and possible ineffective drainage result with high recurrence rate in percutaneous approach, recently, endoscopic method has become a new alternative route and the most preference method nowadays [12].

The first report was published by Sahel et al. in 19 patients with chronic pancreatitis [13]. The complications occurred in four patients (bleeding in two patients, and two perforations). Another pioneer study by Cremer et al. also showed high success rate for endoscopic cystoduodenostomy (ECD) and 100% for endoscopic cystogastrostomy (ECG) [14]. However, both studies were performed in small sample size. Study by Weckman et al. in larger study subjects within 6 years period showed 86.1% success rate for endoscopic management in PPC patients with around 13.9% needing surgical intervention due to unsuccessful therapeutic endoscopy [15].

More studies have been conducted regarding endoscopic transpapillary stenting for pancreatic duct (PD) leak or disruption causing PPC or fistula, and also endoscopic management in WON. First, study by Catalano et al. performing endoscopic cystenterostomy in 8 of 21 PPC patients with duct strictures was successful in all cases [16]. In the recent study of transpapillary management route by Brennan et al., where it only included 30 patients with the indications of PD stenting were PPC, pancreatic ascites, pancreatic duct leak, and fistula, the follow-up success rate after PD stenting for pancreatic duct rupture was 88%, while for pseudocyst, it was 63% [17]. In the WON study, endoscopic treatment was performed in 101 patients. The therapeutic success rate was 98.02%; whereas, long-term follow-up success rate was 96.04% in patients with symptomatic WON [18].

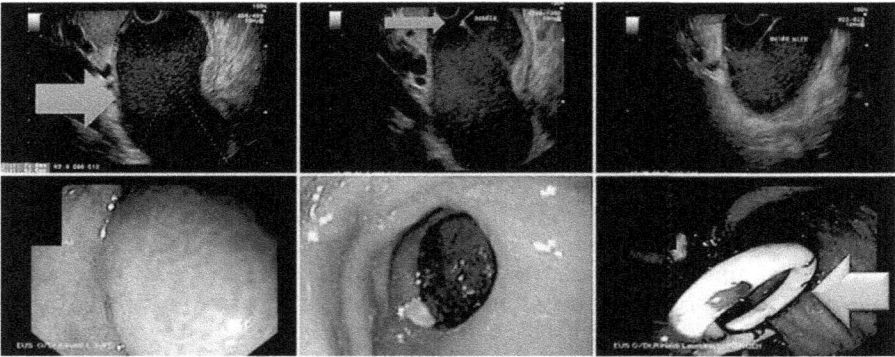

Figure 2.
Patient with pancreatic pseudocyst and gastric outlet obstruction [6].

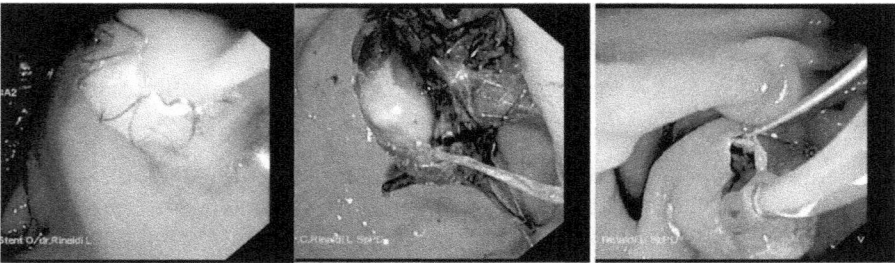

Figure 3.
Patient with infected pancreatic pseudocyst and biliary obstruction (Courtesy: Dr. Cosmas Rinaldi A. Lesmana).

The clinical decision when to intervene the PFC is usually based on comprehensive clinical and imaging evaluation. Gastric outlet obstruction or biliary obstruction needs to be managed as soon as possible (**Figure 2**). It can be recognized early through the clinical symptoms such as abdominal pain, vomiting, weight loss, early satiety, or even jaundice. Infected PPC is one of the absolute indications for drainage procedure (**Figure 3**). Imaging evaluation as well as the fluoroscopy-guided or transabdominal-guided endoscopic management is considered as an important thing, especially in non-bulging PPC [19].

Nowadays, endoscopic ultrasound (EUS) has replaced the traditional way to do the drainage procedure. Through EUS examination, it is easy to evaluate non-bulging PFC as well as other factors, such as the puncture site with large vessels avoidance, accurate fluid aspiration with the wall evaluation, and pancreatic duct connection. Defining the characteristics of each PFC type can also be easily done through EUS examination as the location and the size of the PFC, including the solid material, the wall, and the border, can be scored. It can also evaluate the bile duct under direct visualization [20].

The indication for endoscopic management is usually based on the patient's symptoms, the resolution or severity of infections, and the size of the cyst. Another consideration involves the cyst wall maturity. Usually, the right time to perform endoscopic intervention is after 4 weeks as it allowed better encapsulation. Recent systematic review, comparing percutaneous, surgical, and endoscopic methods in managing PPC, shows that endoscopic management using EUS reduced the length of hospital admission time, cost, and improved patient's quality of life [21, 22].

4. Endoscopic ultrasound-guided pancreatic fluid collection drainage: technical review

There are two options of endoscopic drainage method, which are transmural, transpapillary, or even combining these two techniques. In the pseudocyst case, endoscopic ultrasound (EUS) has been widely used for transmural drainage with previous evaluation where direct visualization of cystic lesions through the gastro-intestinal (GI) lumen can be easily performed. It has become the most important tool in the management for pancreatic cyst, especially to differentiate benign from malignant condition. However, other than anatomic factor, the presence of ductal communication is also an important factor to decide which route is better to perform. In the WON case, the principle is the same; however, the fluid collection resolution after 72 h is the main consideration for more aggressive endoscopic intervention, which is known as EUS-guided transmural necrosectomy procedure. The drainage procedure can be done either with transpapillary or transmural approach. The needle puncture is performed using 19-G FNA needle. After the tip of the needle entering the cyst cavity, the needle sheath can be left inside by pulling out the needle and the guide wire was inserted through the needle sheath until it is coiled up. Then, the sheath was pulled out with maintaining the wire inside the cyst cavity. The dilatation process will further be performed either with dilator or 5 or 6-fr cystotome to make a larger fistula. Finally, the stent is inserted through the fistula track (plastic or metallic stent) [23–26].

5. Endoscopic management: metal vs. plastic stent

There are two types of stents that are usually used in the management of PPC: metal stent and double pigtail plastic stent. There have been some concerns about using the plastic stents, which are possible for re-intervention due to ineffective drainage, longer procedure time regarding the need of two plastic stents place-ment, or even the risk of leakage. However, some studies have shown that plastic stent success rate for PPC drainage ranges from 84 to 94%, but the success rate was found to be lower in few studies when managing WON cases [27–29]. One of the studies by Bang et al. showed that there was no difference for the treatment success between 7 and 10 Fr plastic stents, and even only one plastic stent placement when compared to more than one plastic stents. Another consideration need to be put in clinical practice is the cost, where it would be cheaper to use the plastic stent [30]. Recent meta-analysis study showed that there was a higher clinical success rate (OR 3.39, 95% CI 1.35–21.19) and lower adverse events (OR 0.37, 95% CI 0.21–0.66) in the metal stent studies. The concern is regarding adverse events, such as bleeding, perforation, and stent migration. Fully covered metallic stent (FCMS) might be considered better in bleeding prevention due to the tamponade direct effect from the stent. In the subgroup analysis, even though the success rate in the metal stent group was 98.3%, however, the success rate in the plastic stent group also more than 90%. The success rate in the plastic group was below than 90% only in the WON group, where the metal stent group has still more than 90% success rate [31]. Another development in the stent evolution, lumen apposing metal stent (LAMS) development where this stent is used not only for endoscopic drainage procedure, but also for endoscopic necrosectomy procedure. This stent has also advantage in migration prevention when compared to FCMS [32–35].

Until now, there are still debates and conflicting data with regard to the use of type of the stents. However, even though technically there is no significant differ-ence between placing metal stent versus plastic stent, every type of case need to be decided individually as the cost issue, stent availability, PFC type, and possible complications are still important things for clinical consideration.

6. Conclusions

Acute pancreatitis with pancreatic fluid collection (PFC) is a challenging condition in the field of gastroenterology as it would need good comprehensive clinical assessment and good timing to decide when to intervene. Transmural approach through endoscopic procedure has replaced percutaneous or surgical approach to manage pancreatic pseudocyst. The use of metal stent seemed to be superior than the plastic stent for PFC drainage, however, it would be depending on the cost, availability, and the type of PFC.

Author details

Cosmas Rinaldi Adithya Lesmana[1,2*], Laurentius Adrianto Lesmana[1] and Khek Yu Ho[3]

1 Digestive Disease and GI Oncology Center, Medistra Hospital, Jakarta, Indonesia

2 Department of Internal Medicine, Hepatobiliary Division, Dr. Cipto Mangunkusumo Hospital, Universitas Indonesia, Jakarta, Indonesia

3 Department of Medicine, National University Singapore, Singapore

*Address all correspondence to: medicaldr2001id@yahoo.com

IntechOpen

References

[1] Quinland JD. Acute pancreatitis. American Family Physician. 2014;**90**(9):632-639

[2] Ballie J. Pancreatic pseudocysts (part I). Gastrointestinal Endoscopy. 2004;**59**:873-879

[3] Cui ML, Kim KH, Kim HG, et al. Incidence, risk factors and clinical course of pancreatic fluid collections in acute pancreatitis. Digestive Diseases and Sciences. 2014;**59**:1055-1062

[4] Holt BA, Varadarajulu S. The endoscopic management of pancreatic pseudocysts. Gastrointestinal Endoscopy. 2015;**81**(4):804-812

[5] Giovannini M. What is the best endoscopic treatment for pancreatic pseudocysts? Gastrointestinal Endoscopy. 2007;**65**(4):620-623

[6] Lesmana CRA, Gani RA, Hasan I, Sulaiman AS, Lesmana LA. Case Reports in Gastroenterology. Therapeutic Interventional Endoscopic Ultrasound Based on Rare Cases in Indonesia: A Single-Center Experience in Unselected patients. 2017;**11**(1):72-77

[7] ASGE Standards of Practice committee, Jacobson BC, Baron TH, Adler DG, et al. ASGE guideline: The role of endoscopy in the diagnosis and the management of cystic lesions and inflammatory fluid collections of the pancreas. Gastrointestinal Endoscopy. 2005;**61**:363-370

[8] Shah AP, Mourad MM, Bramhall SR. Acute pancreatitis: Current perspectives on diagnosis and management. The Journal of Inflammation Research. 2018;**11**:77-85

[9] Banks PA, Bollen TL, Dervenis C, et al. Classification of acute pancreatitis—2012: Revision of the Atlanta classification and definitions by international consensus. Gut. 2013;**62**:102-111

[10] Toouli J, Brooke-Smith M, Bassi C, et al. Guidelines for the management of acute pancreatitis. Journal of Gastroenterology and Hepatology. 2002;**17**:515-539

[11] Foster BR, Jensesn KK, Bakis G, Shaaban AM, Coakley FV. Revised atlanta classification for acute pancreatitis: A pictorial essay. RadioGraphics. 2016;**36**:675-687

[12] Turkvatan A, Erden A, Secil M, et al. Fluid collections associated with acute pancreatitis: A pictorial essay. Canadian Association of Radiologists Journal. 2014;**65**:260-266

[13] Tyberg A, Karia K, Gabr M, et al. Management of pancreatic fluid collections: A comprehensive review of the literature. World Journal of Gastroenterology. 2016;**22**(7):2256-2270

[14] Ng PY, Rasmussen DN, Vilmann P, et al. Endoscopic ultrasound-guided drainage of pancreatic pseudocysts: Medium-term assessment of outcomes and complications. Endoscopic Ultrasound. 2013;**2**(4):199-203

[15] Sahel J, Bastid C, Pellat B, et al. Endoscopic cystoduodenostomy of cysts of chronic calcifying pancreatitis: A report of 20 cases. Pancreas. 1987;**2**:447-453

[16] Cremer M, Deviere J, Engelhom L. Endoscopic management of cysts and pseudocysts in chronic pancreatitis: Long-term follow up after 7 years of experience. Gastrointestinal Endoscopy. 1989;**35**:1-9

[17] Weckman L, Kylanpaa ML, Puolakkainen P, et al. Endoscopic treatment of pancreatic pseudocysts. Surgical Endoscopy. 2006;**20**:603-607. Epub: January 19, 2006

[18] Catalano MF, Geenen JE, Schmalz MJ, et al. Treatment of pancreatic pseudocysts with ductal communication by transpapillary pancreatic duct endoprosthesis. Gastrointestinal Endoscopy. 1995;**42**:214-218

[19] Brennan PM, Stefaniak T, Palmer KR, et al. Endoscopic transpapillary stenting of pancreatic duct disruption. Digestive Surgery. 2006;**23**:250-254

[20] Nabi Z, Basha J, Reddy DN. Endoscopic management of pancreatic fluid collections-revisited. World Journal of Gastroenterology. 2017;**23**(15):2660-2672

[21] Alali A, Mosko J, May G, Teshima C. Endoscopic ultrasound-guided management of pancreatic fluid collections: Update and review of the literature. Clinical Endoscopy. 2017;**50**:117-125

[22] Jagielski M, Smoczynski M, Jablonska A, Adrych K. The development of endoscopic techniques for treatment of walled-off pancreatic necrosis: A single-center experience. Gastroenterology Research and Practice. 2018:8149410. DOI: 10.1155/2018/8149410

[23] Dupuis CS, Baptista V, Whalen G, et al. Diagnosis and management of acute pancreatitis and its complications. Gastrointestinal Intervention. 2013;**2**:36-46

[24] Teoh AYB, Dhir V, Jin ZD, et al. Systematic review comparing endoscopic, percutaneous and surgical pancreatic pseudocyst drainage. The World Journal of Gastrointestinal Endoscopy. 2016;**8**(6):310-318

[25] Law R, Baron TH. Endoscopic management of pancreatic pseudocysts and necrosis. Expert Review of Gastroenterology & Hepatology.

Feb 2014;**9**(2):167-175. DOI: 10.1586/17474124.2014.943186

[26] Saftoiu A, Vilmann A, Vilmann P. Endoscopic ultrasound-guided drainage of pancreatic pseudocysts. Endoscopy Ultrasound. 2015;**4**:319-323

[27] Yusuf TE, Baron TH. Endoscopic transmural drainage of pancreatic pseudocysts: Results of a national and an international survey of ASGE members. Gastrointestinal Endoscopy. 2006;**63**:223-227

[28] Samuelson AL, Shah RJ. Endoscopic management of pancreatic pseudocysts. Gastroenterology Clinics of North America. 2012;**41**:47-62. DOI: 10.1016/j.gtc.2011.12.007

[29] Muthusamy VR, Chandrasekhara V, Acosta RD, et al. The role of endoscopy in the diagnosis and treatment of inflammatory pancreatic fluid collections. Gastrointestinal Endoscopy. 2016;**83**(3):481-488

[30] Yasuda I. Endoscopic necrosectomy for infected pancreatic necrosis. Gastrointestinal Intervention. 2012;**1**:36-39

[31] Bang JY, Varadarajulu S. Metal versus plastic stent for transmural drainage of pancreatic fluid collections. Clinical Endoscopy. 2013;**46**:500-502

[32] Yoon SB, Lee IS, Choi MG. Metal versus plastic stents for drainage of pancreatic fluid collection: A meta-analysis. United European Gastroenterology Journal. 2018;**6**(5):729-738

[33] Bugiantella W, Rondelli F, Boni M, et al. Necrotizing pancreatitis: A review of the interventions. The International Journal of Surgery. 2016;**28**:S163-S171

[34] Jurgensen C, Arlt A, Neser F, et al. Endoscopic ultrasound criteria to predict the need for intervention in pancreatic necrosis. BMC Gastroenterology. 2012;**12**:48

[35] Antillon MR, Bechtold ML, Bartalos CR, et al. Transgastric endoscopic necrosectomy with temporary metallic esophageal stent placement for the treatment of infected pancreatic necrosis (with video). Gastrointestinal Endoscopy. 2009;**69**(1):178-180

Up-To-Date View on the Clinical Manifestations and Complications of Chronic Pancreatitis

Mila Dimitrova Kovacheva-Slavova, Plamen Georgiev Getsov,
Georgi Borislavov Vladimirov
and Borislav Georgiev Vladimirov

Abstract

Chronic pancreatitis is an inflammatory disease that causes irreversible anatomical changes including infiltration of inflammatory cells, fibrosis and pancreatic calcification with destruction of the structure of the gland, leading to abdominal pain, endocrine and exocrine dysfunction. Pancreatic exocrine insufficiency (PEI) prevalence in chronic pancreatitis varies between 40 and 94%. PEI is diagnosed by direct and indirect tests. Nutritional status is assessed by anthropometric indicators; laboratory tests—hemoglobin, plasma proteins (albumin, prealbumin, retinol-binding protein, transferrin), fat-soluble vitamins A, D, E, K; micronutrients. Pancreatic enzyme replacement therapy (PERT) is a fundamental part of PEI treatment. An optimal PERT could prevent serious PEI complications such as metabolic bone disease, adverse cardiovascular events, cachexia, poor quality of life and mortality. A periodic screening for PEI complications with a respect to their primary and secondary prophylaxis is mandatory. Diabetes mellitus secondary to pancreatic disease is defined as pancreatogenic diabetes or type 3c diabetes mellitus. Patients with chronic pancreatitis are at increased risk for pancreatic cancer influenced by smoking, alcohol abuse, chronic inflammation and pancreatic stellate cells over-proliferation. However, chronic pancreatitis could be further complicated with splenic vein thrombosis, pseudocysts, duodenal or biliary obstruction, pseudoaneurysm and pancreatic duct stones which might require endoscopic or surgical treatment.

Keywords: chronic pancreatitis, pancreatic exocrine insufficiency, enzyme replacement therapy, pancreatogenic diabetes, pseudocysts, splenic vein thrombosis, duodenal or biliary obstruction, pseudoaneurysm, pancreatic duct stones

1. Introduction

Chronic pancreatitis (CP) is an inflammatory disease that causes irreversible anatomical changes and damage including infiltration of inflammatory cells, fibrotic processes and calcifications formation with destruction of the gland structure and thus affects normal nutrients digestion and absorption. The clinically early phase is characterized by pain and recurrent acute pancreatitis episodes and complications, and the late phase by exo- and/or endocrine insufficiency. In 2016, a new definition of CP was proposed, according to which CP is a fibro-inflammatory syndrome, affecting people with genetic, environmental and/or other risk factors, resulting in a persistent pathological response as a result of parenchymal injury or stress. In addition, some of the following features of advanced CP may be present in each patient: pancreatic atrophy, fibrosis, pain syndrome, ductal stricture, calcifications, pancreatic exocrine/endocrine insufficiency and dysplasia. The frequency of CP per year in the European population is 5–10/100,000. Alcohol abuse is the most observed cause. Recurrent episodes of acute pancreatitis and heredity as a contributing factor may result into CP development [1–7].

Pain is the most frequent symptom in CP patients, leading to quality of life impairment. It pathogenesis is still poorly understood. Multimodal approach, including lifestyle changes, medical therapy, pancreatic endoscopic and surgical procedures, and other non-pharmacological options are recommended [8, 9].

The pancreatic enzymes lipase, amylase, trypsin and chymotrypsin, released predominantly by the duodenal mucosa exposure of nutrients—especially lipids, are at a great importance for the macronutrient digestion. Their secretion comprises the following three phases—maximum, stable and basic secretion. Pancreatic enzymes amount and action duration depend on the caloric content maldigestion, the food type and its physical properties [1, 6, 7, 10, 11].

Pancreatic exocrine insufficiency (PEI) due to a progressive loss of acinar cells is a functional limitation of pancreatic enzyme and bicarbonate secretion, regardless its etiology, leading to digestive process deficiency. Main pathological mechanisms in adults are (1) Insufficient pancreatic secretory capacity, (2) Decreased gland stimulation, (3) Impaired enzymes release in the duodenum. The causes are divided into primary (chronic pancreatitis, cystic fibrosis, pancreatic agenesia, congenital pancreatic hypoplasia, Shwachman-Diamond syndrome, Johanson-Blizzard syndrome, pancreatic lipomatosis or atrophy, isolated lipase or co-lipase deficiency, pancreatic carcinoma, pancreatic resection) and secondary (reduced cholecystokinin releasing, somatostatinoma or exogenous administration of somatostatin, gastrinoma, (sub) total gastrectomy, resections and Billroth II anastomosis, periampullary tumors) [11–15].

Although not studied in-depth, the reported prevalence of PEI in patients with CP varies widely between 40 and 94%. The onset of PEI depends on the CP etiology and is about 10–15 years (5–6 years for alcoholic CP) after initiating the pathological CP processes, which is explained by the large functional reserve capacity. Decompensation occurs when the enzyme secretion is reduced by 90–95%. However, in some patients PEI symptoms such as malnutrition and/or abdominal symptoms (diarrhea, flatulence, pain), steatorrhea, body weight loss are first appearance of the disease [1, 7, 16–18].

Although steatorrhea is a typical symptom of a severe PEI, no clinical symptom unambiguously proves or excludes PEI. Steatorrhea may be absent or caused by pancreatic duct obstruction, low duodenal pH, decreased contact time due to increased motility, small intestinal bacterial overgrowth. Fat-soluble vitamin insufficiency, protein malnutrition, increased risk of osteoporosis and fractures, life-threatening complications such as cardiovascular events are further PEI complications [2, 5, 19–22].

An up-to-date assessment of pancreatic exocrine function allows diagnosis of PEI, initiation of pancreatic enzyme replacement therapy (PERT) and its monitoring. Pancreatic exocrine secretion can be assessed by direct and indirect methods. Direct tests are based on determination of volume, bicarbonates and/or enzymes in the stimulated pancreatic gland by intravenous administration of hormones or their peptide analogs. These methods are invasive because duodenal intubation and a duodenal juice sample are required. Most indirect methods, which evaluate either the digestive ability of the pancreas or the pancreatic secretion by quantification of pancreatic enzymes, are non-invasive, but some require blood sampling and are then considered invasive. The clinical benefit of each method is based on diagnostic accuracy, relevance in clinical practice and cost [20, 23–25].

Pancreatic enzyme replacement therapy is an essential part of PEI treatment. Nowadays a majority of patients with PEI might be asymptomatic, receiving none or suboptimal PERT. They are at increased risk of PEI complications and impaired quality of life. Patients' compliance should be ensured. Periodical monitoring of PERT by nutritional assessment and BMI is mandatory with a respect to primary and secondary prophylaxis of risk factors [1, 6, 18, 26–30].

Pancreatogenic diabetes or type 3c diabetes mellitus develops secondary to pancreatic disease. Recently, DM type 3c is a more recognizable entity due to new proposed criteria. It is a complex disease, further complicated by the presence of comorbidities such as maldigestion and accompanying malnutrition. Metformin is a treatment of choice. Annually screening for type 3c DM by fasting glucose levels and HbA1c is of a great importance in patients with CP regardless the grade of pathological structural changes [17, 18, 20, 31, 32].

Many studies are conducted to demonstrate the association between CP with tropical and hereditary etiology and DM with pancreatic cancer development. The pathogenesis of malignant transformation on the basis of CP remains unclear. Biomarkers and imaging modalities are used to distinguish inflammation form neoplasia [33, 34].

The management of the miscellaneous CP complications pseudocysts, splenic vein thrombosis, duodenal and biliary obstruction, pseudoaneurysm, pancreatic calculi consists of their screening and treating [23].

2. Clinical manifestations of chronic pancreatitis and their management

2.1 Abdominal pain

Abdominal pain is a predominant symptom, affecting 80–90% of patients with CP. Pain significantly reduce quality of life. Pathogenesis is still poorly understood. Multifactorial mechanisms are proposed, including inflammation; duct obstruction followed by hypertension and ischemia; neuronal damage—neuropathic and dysfunctional pain due to hypersensitivity, central and spinal nociceptive neurons alterations. Alcohol and tobacco have contributing role for pain exacerbation. Pancreatic pain covers the characteristics of visceral pain—diffuse severe dull persistent pain, usually with epigastrium location and further radiation to the back, left or right hypochondria. Pain is not necessarily linked to a new acute episode and often worsens with food intake. Pain could be recurrent, during acute episodes and prolonged. Questionnaire scales could be used for pain characterization: Izbicki pain score, brief pain inventory (validated for CP), quantitative sensory testing. According to newest guidelines a multi-modal approach, including lifestyle changes, medical therapy and non-pharmacological approaches, is recommended. Alcohol and tobacco cessation should be advised in all patients. PERT could release pain in patients with ductal obstruction as oral enzymes reduce cholecystokinin levels and therefore decrease pancreatic juice secretion, leading otherwise to duct hypertension. A combination of antioxidants is useful to reduce the oxidative stress and damage. According to the published in 1986 WHO stepwise analgesic's approach is recommended. Simple analgesics (Paracetamol, NSAIDs, Aspirin) are first-line drugs with Paracetamol being the preferable one. If no pain relief is achieved, weak opioids (Tramadol), strong opioids (Morphine, Oxycodone), gabapentinoids (Pregabalin), antidepressants or *N*-methyl-d-aspartate receptor antagonists (Ketamine) could be used. Endoscopic treatment with or without Extracorporeal Shock Wave Lithotripsy has a beneficial role in cases with duct obstruction (see below). If endoscopic treatment is ineffective, surgery procedures (drainage, partial or total resection) are indicated. Better results are observed, when applied in early stages of CP and in patients with no opioids requirements. Other non-pharmacological options in selected patients include bilateral thoracoscopic splanchnicectomy, celiac plexus blocks and splanchnic nerve ablation, spinal cord stimulation, transcranial magnetic stimulation, psychological therapies [8, 9].

2.2 Pancreatic exocrine insufficiency

2.2.1 Pancreatic exocrine insufficiency assessment by direct functional tests

2.2.1.1 Secretin stimulation test

Hormonal stimulation tests are considered to be the most sensitive and specific tests that investigate pancreatic function, including chronic pancreatitis. The test, introduced by Dreiling in 1948, is based on the physiological pancreatic stimulation by secretin with release of water and bicarbonates from the centroacinar and ductal cells. The volume of the duodenum aspiration and bicarbonate concentration are evaluated after double lumen duodenal tube insertion. Standardized ranges, which exclude pancreatic exocrine insufficiency, are: 80–130 mEq/L for peak bicarbonate concentration; 10.1–37.0 mEq/h bicarbonate output, and volume 1.5–5.7 mL/kg for volume/kg. The patient is most likely to suffer from CP if the peak bicarbonate concentration is less than 80 mEq/L. The sensitivity of the test ranges between 60 and 94% and the specificity between 67 and 95%. In a growing number of publications, the use of secretin in the course of other techniques (secretin-enhanced MRCP or endoscopic secretin testing) demonstrates the ability for evaluation of minimal structural changes in the pancreas, in contrast to standard imaging methods which fail to diagnose them [35–38].

2.2.1.2 Cholecystokinin stimulation testing

The classical cholecystokinin stimulation test was developed and first used in the Mayo Clinic. The test measures the enzyme output. Cholecystokinin is given as a continuous infusion of 40 ng/kg/h, but can also be administered as a bolus. Cholecystokinin increases bile secretion in the duodenum during the first 20–40 min after administration, and as a result, the measurement of pancreatic secretion might be affected. The cholecystokinin test disadvantages are as follows: a need for simultaneous gastric and duodenal juices collection during intubation, duodenal perfusion of mannitol and polyethylene glycol solution, delayed stomach emptying, mediation of pain, symptoms of nausea and vomiting most probably due to blood–brain barrier passage [35, 39–43].

2.2.1.3 Secretin-cholecystokinin testing

The combined secretin-cholecystokinin stimulation testing, also called the secretin-pancreozymin test, allows the simultaneous measurement of secretion of both bicarbonate and enzyme by the pancreatic gland. However, cholecystokinin may be administered before or after secretion as long as there is no international standard for test performing and it seems to play insignificant role for diagnostic accuracy. Like the classic cholecystokinin test, it increases the secretion of bile in the duodenum [24, 35, 44].

2.2.1.4 Endoscopic testing

After introducing the idea of obtaining pure pancreatic juice during ERCP in 1982, the technique was adopted and modified by the Japanese pancreatic group and the Cleveland Clinic researchers. The pancreatic fluid collected during ERCP has a higher bicarbonate concentration compared with the classic secretin test (130 mEq/L for healthy subjects and less than 105 mEq/L for CP) and is not contaminated with bile and duodenal content. The drawbacks of the method are the potential ERCP complications, the relatively short time for sample collection—15 min and the need for sedation, which can affect pancreatic secretion. Therefore, the collection of duodenal juice after secretin with or without cholecystokinin stimulation during a standard endoscopic procedure with a tube placed in the endoscope biopsy canal was developed as a comparable alternative. The peak of bicarbonate concentration and the lipolytic activity in the duodenal juice are significantly lower in patients with CP. However, experts find bicarbonate and enzyme output to be more reliable markers for exocrine pancreatic function. Due to its nature—invasiveness, labor intensity, length of procedure (endoscope placement in the duodenum for 1 h) and price, the use of endoscopic tests is limited to some specialized centers, so they are not widely used in everyday practice [24, 39, 45].

2.2.1.5 Secretin-enhanced MRCP (s-MRCP)

Secretin-enhanced MRCP becomes more and more interesting as a method of visualization and morphological assessment of the pancreatic structure, as well as for quantitative assessment of various aspects of pancreatic exocrine function. The magnetic resonance technique has a number of advantages: lack of invasiveness, safety, possibility of three-dimensional reconstruction. The method is costly and is currently limited to large centers, where it is often used in combination with other tests. Its sensitivity is about 90% and is a reliable method for diagnosis of CP in an early stage. In CP, fibrous tissue gradually replaces the glandular elements in the pancreas. This process is reflected in the s-MRCP through characteristic changes in the major pancreatic duct (presence or absence of dilated main pancreatic duct >1 mm), peripheral branches (the presence or absence of dilated peripheral branches) and the volume of pancreatic secretion. The method enables the diagnosis of pancreatic divisum, pseudocysts, ductal disruption resulting from pancreatic necrosis or trauma. For the pancreatic functional evaluation a semiquantitative assessment of the duodenal filling with pancreatic juice at 10th min after secretin application is performed by the following criteria: grade 0-missing duodenal filling; grade 1-only bulbus duodeni filling; grade 2-filling up to genu inferior duodeni; grade 3-fluid filling after genu inferior duodeni. Grade 0–2 is assumed to demonstrate reduced exocrine function. During S-MRCP volume of pancreatic output is predominantly measured. That is why sphincter of Oddi spasm or obstructive lesions may lead to false CP diagnosis. Because of the technique performance and duration the sensitivity could be reduced [35, 46–51].

2.2.2 Pancreatic exocrine insufficiency assessment by indirect functional tests

Indirect pancreatic tests are available in clinical practice and are therefore more common. Indirect tests assess pancreatic exocrine function by quantifying pancreatic digestive ability or pancreatic enzyme levels in feces. The sensitivity and specificity of these indirect tests are variable and lower than the direct ones especially in mild and moderate PEI. From a methodological point of view, tests can be classified as oral and fecal tests.

In the oral tests, the substrate is given per os along with test meal. Pancreatic enzymes hydrolyze the substrate in the duodenum, and released metabolites are absorbed from the intestine, metabolized in the liver and therefore they can be measured in serum, urine or exhaled air. Various extrapancreatic causes could limit the accuracy of oral pancreatic tests, mainly by interfering with normal digestion: reduced gastric emptying, biliary secretion and/or intestinal absorption due to intestinal disease. Impaired gastric emptying may be affected by the administration of metoclopramide or another prokinetic (cisapride, domperidone etc.) [24, 35].

2.2.2.1 ^{13}C-mixed triglycerides breath test

The first oral test for fat malabsorption assessment is based on the use of radioactive iodine ^{131}triolein as a substrate. Modern oral tests use non-radioactive substrates the mixed triglyceride test ^{13}C-MTG-breath test, cholesteryl ^{13}C-octanoate, ^{13}C-hyolein and ^{13}C-triolein. Most commonly used and with the most optimal substrate is the only one optimized so far ^{13}C-MTG breath test, which was introduced into clinical practice by Vantrappen et al. in 1989 and develops as a simple alternative to fecal fat quantification. The test directly measures clinically the most significant effect of exocrine pancreatic function: degradation of triglycerides. Following the already explained metabolic pathway of the labeled substrate in oral tests, ^{13}CO$_2$ is released and eliminated together with the exhaled air and measured by near-infrared analysis or mass spectrometry. Patients with PEI have decreased lipase activity, which can be detected by reduced elimination of ^{13}CO$_2$ in the exhaled air. The ^{13}C-MTG breath test sensitivity for PEI verification is higher than 90%. The current mostly adopted and used protocol is the one developed by Domínguez-Muñoz et al. PEI is diagnosed if values are below 29%. The ^{13}C-MTG breath test is an easy, non-invasive and accurate method of PEI diagnosis. The test is easily applicable in clinical practice and can be repeated as often as necessary. It is also used to monitor the enzyme replacement therapy [24, 52–56].

Fecal tests are based on the quantification of pancreatic enzyme concentration (fecal elastase-1) or activity (chymotrypsin) in feces. Enzymes are deactivated and diluted or concentrated during the intestinal passage, which should be taken into account when interpreting the results [24, 35].

2.2.2.2 Fecal chymotrypsin activity

The test is based on the determination of chymotrypsin activity in a single fecal sample. Fecal chymotrypsin activity lower than 3 U/g is indicative of PEI, but the sensitivity of the test is low. The test is normal in cases of mild CP and in about half of cases with moderate or severe pancreatitis. Significant disadvantages of the test are partial enzyme inactivation during gastrointestinal passage; reduced activity in patients with diarrhea. Quantitative determination of chymotrypsin in feces is an accessible way to assess patient complicity according to the taken replacement therapy as fecal chymotrypsin activity should be significantly increased if oral therapy is administered correctly [24, 35, 57].

2.2.2.3 Fecal elastase-1

The protease elastase represents about 6% of the pancreatic enzyme secretion. Determination of Fecal Elastase-1 (FE-1) is the most common PEI screening test as the enzyme is stable during passage through the gastrointestinal tract, its levels correlate with the secreted amount of the pancreas and the direct functional assays. Even though the determination of FE-1 does not offer a significant advantage over other indirect functional tests, its easy conduction makes it a first step pancreatic function screening tool. FE-1 is determined by monoclonal or polyclonal antibodies ELISA tests. The advantage of monoclonal antibody test is its accuracy during enzyme replacement therapy intake. FE-1 concentrations below 200 µg/g feces indicate PEI, and severe PEI is considered if FE-1 is below 100 µg/g (according to some authors below 50 or even 15 µg/g). The specificity of the test is 93%. Diagnostic sensitivity varies between 54 and 63% in mild pancreatic insufficiency and reaches 82–100% in moderate and severe form. Low levels of FE-1 correlate with morphological changes in CP, objectivized by ERCP and MRCP. Determination of FE-1 is very important and useful in children at the age of 2 months with cystic fibrosis. False positive FE-1 results have been reported in the presence of diarrhea, villous atrophy or a strict vegetarian diet prior to testing [24, 35, 57–62].

2.2.2.4 Steatorrhea-based methods

The amount of released fat in the feces indirectly reflects the degree of fat digestion and thus the secretion of pancreatic lipase. The steatorrhea-based methods are divided into: qualitative (direct microscopy of Sudan III stained preparations), semiquantitative (steatocrit and semiquantitative determination by Sudan III staining) and quantitative (coefficient of fat absorption).

A single fecal sample is used for Sudan III staining. The methodology is based on the number and size of fat drops by high-power field (hpf). The accepted normal ranges are the presence of ≤20 fat drops sized 1–4 µm/hpf. Sudan staining has a sensitivity of up to 94% and 95% specificity for the diagnosis of abnormal fat excretion [35, 63].

Steatocrit is a method for semi-quantitative measurement of fats in feces, expressed as a proportion of the fat content of a single centrifuged and homogenized feces sample. The single determination of acid steatocrit (normal values below 10%) has been shown to have 100% sensitivity for steatorrhea detection and 95% specificity when compared to a 72-h quantitative fat assay [64, 65].

The most reliable and recommended steatorrhea detection method is the 72-h chemical analysis using the van de Kamer method. Many technique modifications have been made so far but still the disadvantages to use large amounts of acids and bases, the manual manipulation of the analysis, the need for additional equipment and specially trained staff remain. However, Near-Infrared Reflectance Analysis (NIRA) methodology, based on the relationship between the intensity of the refractive spectrum of the fecal specimen at a specific wave length and the sample composition, is an alternative, that simplifies and aids application of the study in clinical practice [24, 66].

The coefficient of fat absorption (CFA) is used for a better steatorrhea characterization. The CFA is calculated by the following equation: CFA (%) = 100 × [(mean fat value − mean fat in feces)/average fat intake]. In healthy people CFA is usually over 80%. The technique has a number of disadvantages, that reduce its everyday applicability—a standard diet containing 80–120 g of fat daily for five consecutive days, collection of entire amount of feces from the last 3 days of the diet, inconvenience during feces storing in laboratories, low specificity (any other cause of maldigestion or malabsorption can lead to abnormal fecal fat excretion) [35, 67, 68].

2.2.2.5 Serum trypsin

The trypsin test is the only currently functional diagnostic test that can be performed in serum. Low concentrations of less than 20 ng/mL are specific for CP, but are only sensitive to advanced stage of disease. Levels ranged from 20 to 29 are intermediate, but in some cases may point to an early CP. The sensitivity of the method varies with mild and severe stages of the disease and is between 33 and 65% while the specificity is high. Another advantage of trypsin is that levels above 150 ng/mL are indicative of pancreatic inflammation even in the case of normal amylase and lipase levels [69].

2.2.3 Evaluation of nutritional status as a PEI marker

Malnutrition is a major clinical consequence of PEI. Lindkvist et al. studied 114 patients with CP (EUS, MRCP), 33% suffered from PEI according to ^{13}C-MTG breath test. Hemoglobin, albumin, prealbumin and retinol-binding protein (RBP) levels below reference limit, magnesium less than 2.05 mg/dL and HbA1C above the upper reference limit are associated with PEI. A normal panel of these serum nutritional markers excludes PEI with a high negative predictive value. In case of an abnormality, these parameters serve as a marker for initiating PERT. Their follow-up would indicate the need to adjust the dose of PERT [1, 4, 70].

2.2.4 Pancreatic exocrine insufficiency treatment

Fundamental aspects of PEI treatment, ensuring an optimal therapeutic effect, include pancreatic enzyme replacement therapy (PERT), smoking and alcohol consumption cessation, frequent small meals with a normal fats intake, fat-soluble vitamins and a systemic follow-up with respect to BMI and nutritional markers. The main aim of PEI treatment is, while compensating the lack of endogenous enzyme secretion including lipolysis, to avoid malabsorption and steatorrhea, decrease complications severity, and prevent the associated with malnutrition morbidity and mortality as well as disease progression [1, 7, 18, 20, 26, 71, 72].

Pancreatic enzyme preparations are extracts of porcine pancreas (pancrelipase or pancreatin) with main components: lipase, amylase, trypsin and chymotrypsin. Their alternatives are bovine enzymes, lipase of mushroom origin, bacterial lipase and human lipase. The pancreatic digestive enzymes in PERT are administered orally together with the meal to ensure the mixing of pancreatin with the humus [1, 7, 11, 18, 26, 27, 71, 73, 74].

Currently, the main formulations of the enzyme preparations are with immediate release, enteric-coated microspheres and minimicrospheres, enteric-coated microtablets and enteric-coated microspheres with bicarbonate buffer. The most widely used enzyme preparations are administered as acid-resistant enteric-coated minimicrospheres with a pH-related release. Currently, none of the approved enzyme supplements are specifically designed for use through percutaneous gastrostomy. In infants and patients who cannot swallow large capsules, opening the capsules in a small amount of acidic foods is an acceptable way to administer the drug [1, 2, 12, 75–77].

Although not systematically studied in clinical trials, based on recommendations from different national associations the starting dose of PERT ranges between

20,000 to 50,000 IU lipase per main course and half the dose per snacks, which corresponds to about 5–10% of the cumulative lipase activity in the duodenum after normal meal. PERT is well tolerated with no serious adverse events reported. Fibrosing colonopathy is the only serious complication associated with a high PERT dose. Cases of fibrosing colonopathy have been significantly reduced following the recommendation that PERT should not exceed 10,000 IU lipase/kg/day in patients since 1994 [6, 18, 20, 25, 78–82].

Of a great importance is to ensure patient's compliance. If the signs or symptoms of maldigestion persist, the dose of PERT may be increased twice or three times. As e next step for optimal pH release of enzymes and to influence the precipitation of bile acids and prevent lipase degradation, proton pump inhibitors/antacids/H2 blockers/prostaglandin analogs can be added. If PERT results are still insufficient, diagnosis revision is required in respect to concomitant and/or alternative causes for maldigestion (small intestine bacterial overgrowth, biliary salt deficiency, gastric resection, therapy with certain medications (nonsteroidal anti-inflammatory drugs, antacids). Up to 40% of PEI patients with CP have concomitant small intestinal bacterial overgrowth. Import of 35 kcal/kg/day is required as protein intake of 1.0–1.5 g/kg/day is usually sufficient. Small frequent meals (4–8 times/day) are generally more tolerable than high-calorie meals due to the more effective mixing of the enzyme preparations with the humus. In the modern nutritional concept of PEI no fat restrictions are advisable to reduce the risk of weight loss and deficiency of fat-soluble vitamins. In addition, studies show that corresponding substance presence increases the half-life of the enzyme activity in small intestine [1, 5, 6, 18, 20, 25, 27, 73, 83–87].

Oral, enteral and parenteral nutrition are needed in about 10–15, 5 and 1% of patients respectively, usually in case of disease complications (gastric obstruction) prior to surgery or for a short period of time in patients with advanced exocrine insufficiency [4, 20, 25, 79, 88, 89].

Alcohol and tobacco cessation are of a great importance as they are associated with development of pancreatic cancer, acute and chronic pancreatitis, deterioration of pancreatic exocrine function as shown by endoscopic functional tests in CP cases. Earlier development of calcified pancreatitis and diabetes mellitus are observed in patients with prolonged smoking. Physical activity and a healthy life style along with nutritional therapy should be encouraged for optimal outcome [1, 7, 20, 27, 90].

Most leading researchers recommend a reassessment of symptoms, BMI and serum malnutrition tests with long-term normalization of vitamin status for determining success of PEI treatment. In recent years, studies have shown widespread nutritional deficiencies (fat-soluble vitamins, prealbumin, retinol-binding protein (RBP), and magnesium) in patients with PEI with or without symptoms, which are associated with many risk factors, including malabsorption, diabetes mellitus and alcoholism. Protein markers prealbumin and RBP correlate with age, BMI, morphological changes, fat-soluble vitamins, albumin, hemoglobin, magnesium. According to the United European Gastroenterology evidence based guidelines for the diagnosis and therapy of CP (HaPanEU), PERT should be initiated in patients with PEI in the presence of clinical symptoms or nutritional deficiencies. By PERT optimization in patients with suboptimal dosage an improvement in the nutritional markers is observed [1, 7, 18, 20, 25, 26, 72, 79, 91–95].

Deficiency of vitamins A, D, E, K correlates with the severity of steatorrhea in patients with CP and PEI, but can be caused by various mechanisms, including fat malabsorption, suboptimal nutrition, higher losses or requirements, nutrient depletion, antioxidant activity. Vitamin A, D, E and K deficiency are observed in 3, 53, 10 and 63% of patients (Sikkens et al.) with no clinical manifestations of vitamin E deficiency in up to 75% of CP patients. It has been established that the severity of CP (according to the Cambridge classification) correlates with the bone mineral density of the spine and the femoral neck. Patients with CP regardless their exocrine status have more often than expected reduced bone mineral density as shown in a recent meta-analysis: 1 in 4 patients were diagnosed with osteoporosis and 2/3 with osteopathy. Risk factors for fractures include female gender, older patients (the relative risk is higher in younger patients), smoking, alcohol consumption (60–150% greater risk than non-alcoholic CP patients), chronic inflammation, low BMI regardless of bone mineral density. The incidence of fractures after minimal trauma among CP patients is comparable and even higher than in patients with high-risk gastrointestinal diseases (Crohn's disease, cirrhosis, celiac disease, after gastrectomy), for which guidelines for osteoporosis screening exists. The treatment of osteopathy should be carried out in accordance with up-to-date guidelines on the treatment of metabolic bone disease in the general population [2, 14, 16, 27, 28, 59, 65, 96–103].

In addition to bone metabolism, vitamin D is a factor in the development of pancreatic fibrosis and atrophy, cardiovascular and autoimmune diseases, type 1 and 2 diabetes mellitus, and contributes to an increased overall mortality [104, 105].

Due to insufficient protease secretion from the pancreas, vitamin B12 deficiency may occur. Micronutrient deficiencies have been reported as well: zinc (especially in diabetes mellitus), calcium (normal levels in patients receiving PERT), magnesium, thiamine and folic acid, riboflavin, choline, manganese, sulfur, copper and others [106–108].

The assessment of fat-soluble vitamins, minerals and trace elements and bone density should be monitored 1–2 times a year [109].

2.2.5 Cardiovascular risk evaluation

A recent study observed increased mortality in patients with PEI. Patients who died used to have a worse nutritional status. However, an optimal PERT is essential to reduce morbidity and mortality associated with CP. Maldigestion is associated with life-threatening complications such as cardiovascular, cachexia, which are related to low plasma levels of the cardioprotective HDL, apolipoprotein (apo) A-I and lipoprotein A (2). In a recent study in patients with CP who had not received PERT, mean triglyceride levels were found to be significantly higher in patients with PEI than those without PEI. According to randomized clinical trials, mean levels of cholesterol, HDL, LDL and triglycerides in patients with CP and PEI receiving PERT have been reported in reference ranges. Based on American, European and Canadian guidelines, a complex approach, including screening systems, lipid profile, apolipoproteins, is needed to properly assess cardiovascular risk. Apolipoprotein B as part of all atherogenic or potentially atherogenic particles including LDL, VLDL, IDL, lipoprotein (a) (each particle contains 1 molecule of apo B) provides direct measurement of all atherogenic lipoprotein particles in the circulation, which makes apo B more reliable indicator of cardiovascular risk than LDL. Clinical and epidemiological studies confirm that apo B and Apo B/Apo A-I ratio are associated with a worse outcome in patients with cardiovascular diseases and are supposed to predict cardiovascular incidents more accurately than the routinely tested cholesterol, LDL, TC/HDL, non-HDL. The proposed cut-off values for Apo B/ApoA-I ratio predicting high cardiovascular risk (acute myocardial infarction) are 0.9 for men and 0.8 for women. In patients with Apo B/ApoA-I ratio higher than 0.9, higher triglyceride levels and plasma atherogenic index and lower apo E were found. A study demonstrates an increased risk of myocardial infarction using Apo B/Apo A-I ratio in patients with CP [1, 5, 7, 79, 89, 110–131].

Apolipoprotein A, which is the main apolipoprotein associated with HDL, has two forms—apo A-I and apo A-II. The levels of apolipoprotein A-I are strongly related to those of HDL and can serve for plasma HDL level determination. In a recent study, an impaired nutritional status with decreased prealbumin, RBP, hemoglobin, magnesium has been found to significantly relate to low apoA-I and apoA-II levels with a tendency of increased apo B/apo A-I ratio, which does not reach a significant value. Apolipoprotein C-III inhibits the lipolysis of triglyceride-rich lipoproteins and complicates their elimination from the bloodstream. High levels of apolipoprotein C-III are associated with an increased risk of cardiovascular events and atherogenesis. Lower apolipoprotein C-III levels are observed by morphological changes worsening in CP. The metabolic and inflammatory status in patients with CP can be traced with great accuracy by examining a protein panel of retinol binding protein, serum amyloid-alpha, Apo A-II, Apo A-I, Apo C-I, Apo C-II, Apo C-III and prealbumin, which are significantly more reduced than the controls (Hartmann et al.). The observed changes may be associated with underlying malnutrition/cachexia, which phenomena are known in the modulation of the synthesis of acute phase proteins in acute or chronic disease [112, 119, 127, 128, 130, 132–137].

2.3 Pancreatic endocrine insufficiency

In respect to its etiology, the diabetes mellitus (DM), which is caused by pancreatic diseases, is defined by the American Diabetes Association (ADA) and World Health Organization as pancreatogenic diabetes or Type 3c DM and is included in "other specific forms of diabetes" (ADA). About 5–10% of all diabetic patients in Western populations fulfill the criteria for pancreatogenic DM, of which circa 80% have underlying CP. The prevalence and clinical significance of DM secondary to CP has been recently underestimated. The median survival is 8.7 years after diagnosing type 3c DM. Chronic pancreatitis and DM are independent risk factors for pancreatic cancer development. While the presence of anti-insulin antibodies and clinical or biochemical data on insulin resistance are associated with type 1 and 2 DM respectively, the pathogenesis of type 3c DM is very complex. According to the recommendations of Rickels MR et al. from the Pancreas Fest 2012, the following criteria for the diagnosis of type 3c DM were proposed. Major criteria (all must be fulfilled): (1) Pancreatic exocrine insufficiency. (2) Pathological pancreas imaging (EUS, MRI, CT). (3) Lack of type 1 DM associated with the presence of autoantibodies. Minor criteria: (1) Impaired beta-cell function (HOMA-B, C-peptide/glucose ratio). (2) Lack of insulin resistance (HOMA-IR). (3) Invasive secretion disorder (GLP-1, pancreatic polypeptide). (4) Low levels of serum fat-soluble vitamins (A, D, E, K). Because of loss of glucagon response to hypoglycemia and low carbohydrate levels (malabsorption; inadequate food intake due to pain, nausea and/or chronic alcohol abuse), patients with type 3c DM may experience frequent episodes of hypoglycemia, making the glucose control challenging. The course of the disease is further complicated by the presence of comorbidities such as maldigestion and accompanying malnutrition. Metformin, which is recommend as first-line treatment for type 2 DM by ADA and EASD, has been shown to reduce the risk of pancreatic cancer by 70% and the associated mortality, making metformin suitable therapeutic option for type 3c DM patients. The associated with an increased risk of developing pancreatitis as well as numerous gastrointestinal side effects (nausea, delayed gastric emptying, weight loss) GLP-1 analogues and DPP4-inhibitors should be avoided as long as their safety and benefits are proven. Impaired incretin hormone secretion can be normalized by supplementation with pancreatic enzymes, which is reflected in improved insulin secretion and glucose tolerance during meals. Adequate oral enzyme replacement affects steatorrhea, prevents malnutrition and metabolic complications. In patients with severe malnutrition, insulin therapy is a first-line of choice because of the anabolic effect of insulin. The association of low levels of vitamin D and poor glycemic control draws attention to the need to normalize vitamin status in patients with type 3c DM. Diagnosis and monitoring of DM should be consistent with the endocrinology societies guidelines. Annually screening for type 3c DM by fasting glucose and HbA1c is of a great importance in patients with CP regardless the grade of pathological structural changes [18, 20, 25, 31, 32, 122, 138–143].

3. Chronic pancreatitis complications and their management

3.1 Pancreatic cancer

Since the first report by Rocca et al. in 1987 for an increased incidence of pancreatic cancer (PC) in patients with CP, several epidemiological studies have identified that CP, mainly tropical and hereditary pancreatitis, is a major risk factor for pancreatic cancer development. Augustine et al. reported that PC is affecting 8.3% of patients with CP with a roughly 100-fold higher incidence compared to patients without tropical pancreatitis. Younger patients are affected and have a worse outcome. In hereditary CP due to multiple PRSS1 mutations the lifetime risk for PC is 40–55% by the age of 70. Possible explanations for the increased neoplastic transformation risk are the onset of CP at younger age and its long duration. Various risk factors for PC development have been described, of which smoking is the major one. In a recent study, Hao et al. (2017) suggest that age at the onset of CP (hazard ratio, 1.05) and a > 60 pack-year smoking history (hazard ratio, 11.83) are PC risk factors. CP as an inflammatory disease is associated with higher cell turnover with/without DNA damage, progressing to oncogenic mutations in K-ras, p16 and p53 promoting metaplasia and neoplastic degeneration. Another well-known PC risk factor is diabetes mellitus. Ethanol and its metabolites are supposed to activate pancreatic stellate cells over-proliferation. They play a role in tumor progression and chemotherapy resistance. Moreover, cholecystokinin receptors are abnormally over-produced. Clinical features may mimic those of CP in early stages. When symptoms such as obstructive jaundice, pain, weight loss and worsening of diabetes appear, all of which are specific for malignancy, this generally indicates that the disease is at an advanced stage. The most investigated biomarker for malignancy prediction is CA 19–9 with 96.5–100% specificity. Based on metabolic biomarkers, Mayerle et al. (2018) introduce a novel approach for differential diagnose between CP and PC with an accuracy of 90% and a negative predictive value of 99.9%. Other promising markers are plasma micro-RNAs, monoclonal antibody PAM4, CD1D, which require further investigation. For the imaging diagnosis of PC, a CT scan is the technique of choice. Endoscopic ultrasound (EUS) could detect small pancreatic tumors in CP patients at a highest sensitivity compared to the available imaging and has the potential to detect early stage PC. The most appropriate cancer treatment (surgery, chemotherapy, radiation) depends on disease proliferation, defining the cancer as resectable, locally advanced or metastatic [144–149].

3.2 Pseudocysts

Pancreatic pseudocysts are common complication in CP with a frequency of 20–40%. The majority of patients are with alcoholic (70–80%) or idiopathic etiology of CP (6–16%). The outcome of pseudocysts is assessed 6 weeks after acute episode occurring. In 40% of the pseudocysts there is a spontaneous resolution, another 40% of pseudocysts remain asymptomatic and in 20% of pseudocysts complications are observed (infection, rupture, bleeding, splenic vein thrombosis). Treatment is required if patients are symptomatic, if complications or obstruction of the stomach, duodenum or bile duct occur. Drainage of chronic pseudocysts may be performed by surgical, endoscopical or percutaneous approach. In asymptomatic pseudocysts with size above 5 cm, due to high possibility of complications, an endoscopical or surgical treatment is recommended. Percutaneous drainage should be avoided where possible. In chronic pseudocysts the endoscopical procedure is the treatment of choice due to lower mortality rate, improved quality of life and less length of hospitalization stay. Depending on size and localization, two endoscopic techniques are performed. A transpapillary approach should be considered in small pseudocysts with communication with the main pancreatic duct. The transmural approach (cystogastrostomy) is similar to the management of walled-off necrosis. It is more successful under echoendoscopic guidance. Double-pigtail plastic stents for at least 2 months are used for pseudocyst drainage. If a malignant genesis of the pseudocyst is suspected, surgery should follow [148, 150–156].

3.3 Splenic vein thrombosis

In 1920 Hirschfeldt first reported splenic vein thrombosis (SVT) as a pancreatitis consequence. Secondary involvement of the splenic vein endothelium by a nearby inflammation, compression by a pseudocyst or enlarged retroperitoneal/pancreatic lymph nodes or initial injury could result in a splenic vein thrombosis and obstruction. The incidence of SVT in patients with CP is 1.5–41.6%. Sinistral portal hypertension and collateral development resulting in gastric and/or esophageal varices are major risk factor for bleeding. Splenomegaly is reported in 42–54% of patients. Most patients are asymptomatic. Clinical features include gastrointestinal bleeding in 12.3% of cases and abdominal pain. SVT is diagnosed primary by contrast-enhanced CT scan and/or upper endoscopy. Venous phase angiography is the gold standard confirmatory test, which could verify obstruction and collaterals routes. Based on the widely available CT scan most patients nowadays are diagnosed asymptomatic. The SVT management depends on existing symptoms including hypersplenic syndrome and history of variceal bleeding, which might require splenectomy with venous collateral outflow elimination and further variceal decompression. Gastric varices should be treated endoscopically by sclerotherapy, gastric banding [148, 157–162].

3.4 Duodenal obstruction

The duodenal obstruction is a rare complication in CP patients (1%) due to the anatomical relationship between the duodenum and the head of the pancreas. However, when analyzing operated patients with CP, the incidence of duodenal obstruction is higher—12%. Two types of obstruction are observed—transients during acute pancreatitis episodes and fixed by pseudocyst compression (discussed above) or fibrosclerotic process. Paraduodenal or groove pancreatitis is a rare clinic-pathological focal type of CP. The reported incidence of groove pancreatitis in resected CP patients ranges between 2.7 and 24.5%. It was first described by Becker in 1973 as a segmental pancreatitis. In 2004 Adsav and Zamboni unify the previously described terms under paraduodenal pancreatitis. The proposed pathophysiological mechanisms comprise functional/

anatomical obstruction of papilla minor, Brunner's gland hyperplasia around papilla minor, heterotopic intraduodenal pancreatic tissue or ductal variation. Two types paraduodenal pancreatitis are defined–cystic and solid. The cystic type is common with localization in the submucosa or lamina propria. The size may reach 10 cm, resulting in a bile duct obstruction. The solid type is rare and includes sheet-like and mass-like subtypes. According to several retrospective studies, the risk groups for paraduodenal pancreatitis development are middle-aged men with alcohol consumption. Acute manifestation complains include postprandial abdominal pain (90–100%), nausea and vomiting (20%), gastric outlet syndrome. Chronic manifestations are weight loss (90%) and jaundice (20%). Perforation, bleeding, malignant degeneration of heterotopic pancreas are reported rare complications. EUS and MRCP are the preferred imaging methods for diagnostic evaluation. Treatment is based on a stepwise approach: (1) conservative treatment (analgesics, infusions, PPI, PERT, enteral nutrition, somatostatin analogues); (2) endoscopic treatment; (3) surgery (Whipple procedure, pancreaticoduodenectomy, suprapapillar duodenal resection in isolated duodenal dystrophy, palliative gastrojejunostomy) [8, 148, 163–170].

3.5 Biliary obstruction

The incidence of distal common bile duct obstruction in patients with advanced chronic predominantly calcific pancreatitis with frequent acute episodes ranges from 3 to 46%. Pseudocysts are considered more as a risk factor than as a cause. Patients may be asymptomatic or with various spectrum of complains and complications—pain, jaundice (transient or persistent for longer than 1 month), cholangitis and even sepsis, long-term risk of secondary biliary cirrhosis. Hyperbilirubinemia and twofold elevation of alkaline phosphatase levels for more than a month are used as reliable laboratory markers for common bile duct obstruction. CT scan provides information for the structural changes with high specificity and sensitivity. Based on the Caroli and Nora criteria, most patients with common bile duct stricture and CP are classified as type I and III. The treatment of choice depends on presence and severity and duration of symptoms; suspected malignant degeneration. To prevent progression to secondary biliary cirrhosis in patients with progressively increased alkaline phosphatase levels or persistent/with frequent relapses hyperbilirubinemia, endoscopic biliary stenting with self-expanding metal stents or multiple plastic stents or surgical procedures (pancreaticoduodenectomy, choledochojejunostomy, choledochoduodenostomy, hepaticojejunostomy) are required [148, 171–173].

3.6 Pseudoaneurysm

Pancreatic pseudoaneurysm as a rare life-threatening chronic pancreatitis complication occurs in 10% of patients, most often in those with pseudocysts. The pseudoaneurysm represents fibrous tissue containing hematoma and is mainly induced by enzymatic autodigestion or eroding of the nearby vessels, most frequent affecting the splenic artery. Most patients are asymptomatic, however, the first clinical manifestation might be bleeding caused by pseudoaneurysm rupture into gastrointestinal tract or other adjacent anatomic structures—peritoneal cavity, retroperitoneum, biliopancreatic ducts (hemosuccus pancreaticus). Shock and multiorgan failure further complicate the rupture. The mortality rate is about 40% and higher (90–100%) if pseudoaneurysm remains untreated. Worst outcome results have been shown in patients with pseudoaneurysm localization in the pancreas head. Angiography is the diagnostic tool of choice. Patients are nowadays treated surgical, endovascular, by angioembolization and/or by percutaneous ultraso-nographically guided thrombin injection. Treatment in diagnosed asymptomatic patients is recommended [174–179].

3.7 Pancreatic duct stones

In about 50% of patients chronic inflammation, gene predisposition and alcohol intake as a key cause change the pancreatic juice composition with pancreatic stone protein levels reduction, leading to formation of a nucleus with calcium deposi-tion layers and later formation of a stone. The pancreatic duct stones are classified according to their number, localization and density to single or multiple calculi; stones in the pancreatic head, body and/or tail; localized in the main pancreatic duct, side-branches and/or parenchyma; radiopaque positive (the majority of cases), negative or mixed stones. The main pathological consequence is the duct obstruction with upstream dilatation, followed by ductal hypertension, which results in pain episodes, exocrine insufficiency due to reduce pancreatic juice flow into duodenum and impaired quality of life. Pancreatic duct stones are diagnosed by ERCP, CT or MRCP. However, MRCP is superior to ERCP for diagnosis as MRCP is a non-invasive alternative with no complications, providing detailed information about duct system and stone formations. Calculi removal could be performed by extracorporeal shock wave lithotripsy (ESWL), endoscopic techniques and surgery. According to the European Society of Gastrointestinal Endoscopy guidelines, first-line therapy for painful uncomplicated CP is ESWL combined or not with ERCP followed by spontaneous expulsion or endoscopic extraction of less than 3 mm fragments. However, ESWL should be performed in centers with ESWL expertise. Best results from endoscopic techniques are observed in patients with early stages of CP with infrequent pain attacks, when calculi are less than 5 mm and have head localization with upstream main pancreatic duct dilatation. Alcohol and tobacco cessation improve the long-lasting results. Endoscopic techniques include ERCP followed by pancreatic sphincterotomy; stone retrieval with a bal-loon, Dormia basket and/or forceps; dilatation and stent placement; mechanical lithotripsy. Endoscopy procedures together with ESWL improve the success to up to 90%. Direct visualization by pancreatoscopy followed by intraductal lithotripsy (Spyglass system) might be a future procedure of choice but today its use is limited. Surgery should be performed in patients with large or multiple calculi and stric-tures, after unsuccessful prior endoscopy or ESWL procedures, as well as in those with no pain relief [8, 180–183].

4. Quality of life

With disease progression, patients with CP report for impaired overall quality of life. Many studies are conducted to investigate the contributing factors, leading to low QoL. Pain significantly correlates with overall health status, physical and mental subscales. Researchers emphasize the role of severity in contrast to pain frequency and pathophysiology. A large study of Machiado et al., including 1024 CP patients, highlights constant pain as well as inability due to pain, smoking status and concomitant co-morbidities to worsen significantly QoL with negative influ-ence on both physical and mental domains, leading to worsened social and family status and health resource utilization. Other assumed factors, which importance differs among the literature data, are disease duration, young age, women, tobacco and alcohol intake, underweight, pancreatic structural changes DM, PEI, prior endoscopic or surgical treatments. Psychologically conditioned disturbances (depression, anxiety etc.) are linked most often to alcohol abuse and might lead to pain manifestation and impaired QoL. A study, which enrolled non-alcoholic CP patients, significant depressive syndromes were associated with poor QoL. By the newest concepts, the quality of life assessment is an essential part of the monitoring and the outcome in patients with CP. The European Organization for Research and Treatment of Cancer (EORTC QLQ) has developed a quality of life questionnaire, containing 30 questions (EORTC QLQ-C30), including an additional question about steatorrhea. The questionnaire correlates with body weight gain and a reduced number of daily defecations related to malnutrition and maldigestion. The quality of life improved after adequate dosing in both newly diagnosed and patients receiving suboptimal PERT. Later, an additional panel of 26 questions concerning pancreatic cancer patients (PAN26) was developed. In the United European Gastroenterology evidence based guidelines for the diagnosis and therapy of CP (HaPanEU), quality of life including pain should be assessed through validated questionnaires (SF-12, SF-36, EORTC QLQ C-30, GIQLI). However, effort should be point at improvement of variable factors as psychological status, tobacco, alcohol consumption and nutritional deficiencies in respect to improve QoL and further to delay disease progression, using therapeutic education and physical rehabilitation, behavioral support and medication [6, 99, 184–190].

5. Conclusion

Chronic pancreatitis is a progressive fibro-inflammatory syndrome, leading to abdominal pain and later to endocrine and exocrine insufficiency. Patients with CP might suffer a wide variety of complications, including pancreatic cancer, splenic vein thrombosis, pseudocysts, duodenal or biliary obstruction, pancreatic calculi, pseudoaneurysm and cardiovascular events. Proper individual up-to-date approach to diagnosis, treatment and follow-up of patients with CP are of fundamental importance to improve symptoms, detect early risk factors and reduce complications, which are associated with high mortality rate, and ensure better quality of life. Screening strategies development and their introduction into the clinical practice should be encouraged.

Author details

Mila Dimitrova Kovacheva-Slavova[1*], Plamen Georgiev Getsov[2],
Georgi Borislavov Vladimirov[3] and Borislav Georgiev Vladimirov[1]

1 Department of Gastroenterology, University Hospital "Tsaritsa Ioanna-ISUL",
Medical University of Sofia, Sofia, Bulgaria

2 Department of Medical Imaging, University Hospital "Tsaritsa Ioanna-ISUL",
Medical University of Sofia, Sofia, Bulgaria

3 Department of Cardiology, National Heart Hospital, Sofia, Bulgaria

*Address all correspondence to: kovacheva_mila@abv.bg

IntechOpen

References

[1] Lindkvist B. Diagnosis and treatment of pancreatic exocrine insufficiency. World Journal of Gastroenterology. 2013;**19**(42):7258-7266. ISSN: 1007-9327 (print); ISSN: 2219-2840

[2] D'Haese JG, Ceyhan GO, Demir IE, et al. Pancreatic enzyme replacement therapy in patients with exocrine pancreatic insufficiency due to chronic pancreatitis: A 1-year disease management study on symptom control and quality of life. Pancreas. 2014;**43**:834-841

[3] Stevens T, Conwell DL, Zuccaro G. Pathogenesis of chronic pancreatitis: An evidence-based review of past theories and recent developments. The American Journal of Gastroenterology. 2004;**99**:2256-2270. DOI: 10.1111/j.1572-0241.2004.40694.x

[4] Lindkvist B, Phillips ME, Domínguez-Muñoz JE. Clinical, anthropometric and laboratory nutritional markers of pancreatic exocrine insufficiency: Prevalence and diagnostic use. Pancreatology. 2015;**15**(6):589-597. DOI: 10.1016/j.pan.2015.07.001

[5] de la Iglesia-García D, Huang W, Szatmary P, et al. Efficacy of pancreatic enzyme replacement therapy in chronic Pancreatitis: systematic review and meta-analysis. Gut. 2017;**66**:1354-1355

[6] Löhr JM et al. United European Gastroenterology evidence-based guidelines for the diagnosis and therapy of chronic pancreatitis (HaPanEU). United European Gastroenterology Journal;**5**(2):153-199

[7] Braganza JM, Lee SH, McCloy RF, McMahon MJ. Chronic pancreatitis. Lancet. 2011;**377**(9772):1184-1197. DOI: 10.1016/S0140-6736(10)61852-1

[8] Drewes AM, Bouwense SA, Campbell CM, Ceyhan GO, Delhaye MN, Demir IE, et al. Guidelines for the understanding and management of pain in chronic pancreatitis. Pancreatology: Official Journal of the International Association of Pancreatology (IAP). 2017;**17**(5):720-731

[9] Goulden MR. The pain of chronic pancreatitis: A persistent clinical challenge. British Journal of Pain. 2013;**7**(1):8-22

[10] Witt H, Apte MV, Keim V, Wilson JS. Chronic pancreatitis: Challenges and advances in pathogenesis, genetics, diagnosis, and therapy. Gastroenterology. 2007;**132**:1557-1573. DOI: 10.1053/j.gastro.2007.03.001

[11] Krishnamurty DM, Rabiee A, Jagannath SB, Andersen DK. Delayed release pancrelipase for treatment of pancreatic exocrine insufficiency associated with chronic pancreatitis. Therapeutics and Clinical Risk Management. 2009;**5**(3):507-520

[12] Lowe ME. The structure and function of pancreatic enzymes. In: Johnson LR, Alpers DH, Christensen J, Jacobson ED, Walsh JH, editors. Physiology of the Gastrointestinal Tract. Vol. 2. New York: Raven Press; 1994. pp. 1531-1542

[13] Nakajima K, Oshida H, Muneyuki T, Kakei M. Pancrelipase: An evidence-based review of its use for treating pancreatic exocrine insufficiency. Core Evidence. 2012;**7**:77-91

[14] Petersen JM, Forsmark CE. Chronic pancreatitis and maldigestion. Seminars in Gastrointestinal Disease. 2002;**13**:191-199

[15] Sander-Struckmeier S, Beckmann K, Janssen-van Solingen G, et al. Retrospective analysis to investigate the effect of concomitant use of gastric acid-suppressing drugs on the

efficacy and safety of pancrelipase/
pancreatin (CREON(R)) in patients
with pancreatic exocrine insufficiency.
Pancreas. 2013;**42**:983-989

[16] Bruno MJ, Haverkort EB, Tytgat GN,
van Leeuwen DJ. Maldigestion
associated with exocrine pancreatic
insufficiency: Implications of
gastrointestinal physiology and
properties of enzyme preparations for
a cause-related and patient-tailored
treatment. The American Journal of
Gastroenterology. 1995;**90**(9):1383-1393

[17] Czako L, Hegyi P, Rakonczay Z Jr,
Wittmann T, Otsuki M. Interactions
between the endocrine and exocrine
pancreas and their clinical relevance.
Pancreatology. 2009;**9**(4):351-359

[18] de-Madaria E, Abad-González A,
Aparicio JR, Aparisi L, et al.
The Spanish Pancreatic Club's
recommendations for the diagnosis
and treatment of chronic pancreatitis:
Part 2 (treatment). Pancreatology.
2013;**13**(1):18-28

[19] Borgstrom B. Influence of bile salt,
pH, and time on the action of pancreatic
lipase. Journal of Lipid Research.
1964;**5**:522-531

[20] Toouli J, Biankin AV, Oliver MR,
Pearce CB, Wilson JS, Wray NH, et al.
Management of pancreatic exocrine
insufficiency: Australasian pancreatic
club recommendations. The Medical
Journal of Australia. 2010;**193**:461-467

[21] Waljee AK, Dimagno MJ, Wu BU,
Schoenfeld PS, Conwell DL. Systematic
review: Pancreatic enzyme treatment of
malabsorption associated with chronic
pancreatitis. Alimentary Pharmacology
& Therapeutics. 2009;**29**:235-246

[22] Whitcomb DC, Lehman GA,
Vasileva G, et al. Pancrelipase delayed
release capsules (CREON) for exocrine
pancreatic insufficiency due to chronic
pancreatitis or pancreatic surgery: A
double-blind randomized trial. The
American Journal of Gastroenterology.
2010;**105**(10):2276-2286

[23] Ramsey ML, Conwell DL,
Hart PA. Complications of chronic
pancreatitis. Digestive Diseases and
Sciences. 2017;**62**(7):1745-1750

[24] Domínguez-Muñoz JE. Diagnosis of
chronic pancreatitis: Functional testing.
Best Practice & Research. Clinical
Gastroenterology. 2010;**24**(3):233-241

[25] Frulloni L et al. Italian consensus
guidelines for chronic pancreatitis.
Digestive and Liver Disease.
2010;**42**(Suppl 6):S381-S406

[26] Delhaye M, Van Steenbergen W.,
Cesmeli E, Pelckmans P, Putzeys V,
Roeyen G, Berrevoet Ugent F, Scheers I,
Ausloos F, Gast P, et al. Belgian consensus
on chronic pancreatitis in adults and
children: statements on diagnosis and
nutritional, medical, and surgical
treatment Acta Gastro-Enterologica
Belgica. 2014;**77**(1):47-65

[27] Domínguez-Muñoz JE. Pancreatic
enzyme therapy for exocrine pancreatic
insufficiency. Current Gastroenterology
Reports. 2007;**9**:116-122

[28] Sikkens EC, Cahen DL, van Eijck C,
Kuipers EJ, Bruno MJ. Patients with
exocrine insufficiency due to chronic
pancreatitis are undertreated: A
Dutch national survey. Pancreatology.
2012;**12**:71-73

[29] Sikkens EC, Cahen DL, Koch AD,
Braat H, Poley JW, Kuipers EJ, et al.
The prevalence of fat-soluble vitamin
deficiencies and a decreased bone mass
in patients with chronic pancreatitis.
Pancreatology. 2013;**13**(3):238-242. DOI:
10.1016/j.pan.2013.02.008

[30] Nakamura T, Takebe K, Imamura K,
Tando Y, Yamada N, Arai Y, et al. Fat-
soluble vitamins in patients with chronic
pancreatitis (pancreatic insufficiency).

Acta Gastroenterologica Belgica. 1996;**59**:10-14

[31] Ewald N, Raspe A, Kaufmann C, Bretzel RG, Kloer HU, Hardt PD. Determinants of exocrine pancreatic function as measured by fecal elastase-1 concentrations (FEC) in patients with diabetes mellitus. European Journal of Medical Research. 2009;**14**(3):118-122

[32] Hardt PD, Ewald N. Exocrine pancreatic insufficiency in diabetes mellitus: A complication of diabetic neuropathy or a different type of diabetes? Experimental Diabetes Research. 2011;**2011**:761950. DOI: 10.1155/2011/761950

[33] Dhar P, Kalghatgi S, Saraf V. Pancreatic cancer in chronic pancreatitis. Indian Journal of Surgical Oncology. 2015;**6**(1):57-62

[34] Kong X, Sun T, Kong F, Du Y, Li Z. Chronic pancreatitis and pancreatic cancer. Gastrointest Tumors. 2014;**1**(3):123-134

[35] Lieb JG, Draganov PV. Pancreatic function testing: Here to stay for the 21st century. World Journal of Gastroenterology. 2008;**14**(20):3149-3158

[36] Dreiling DA, Hollander F. Studies in pancreatic function; preliminary series of clinical studies with the secretin test. Gastroenterology. 1948;**11**:714-729

[37] Kitagawa M, Naruse S, Ishiguro H, Nakae Y, Kondo T, Hayakawa T. Evaluating exocrine function tests for diagnosing chronic pancreatitis. Pancreas. 1997;**15**:402-408

[38] Steer ML, Waxman I, Freedman S. Chronic pancreatitis. The New England Journal of Medicine. 1995;**332**:1482-1490

[39] Stevens T, Conwell DL, Zuccaro G Jr, et al. A prospective crossover study comparing secretin-stimulated endoscopic and dreiling tube pancreatic function testing in patients evaluated for chronic pancreatitis. Gastrointestinal Endoscopy. 2008;**67**:458-466

[40] Gullo L, Costa PL, Fontana G, Labo G. Investigation of exocrine pancreatic function by continuous infusion of caerulein and secretin in normal subjects and in chronic pancreatitis. Digestion. 1976;**14**:97-107

[41] Schibli S, Corey M, Gaskin KJ, Ellis L, Durie PR. Towards the ideal quantitative pancreatic function test: Analysis of test variables that influence validity. Clinical Gastroenterology and Hepatology. 2006;**4**:90-97

[42] Conwell DL, Zuccaro G, Morrow JB, Van Lente F, Obuchowski N, Vargo JJ, et al. Cholecystokinin-stimulated peak lipase concentration in duodenal drainage fluid: A new pancreatic function test. American Journal of Gastroenterology. 2002;**97**:1392-1397

[43] Conwell DL, Zuccaro G, Morrow JB, et al. Analysis of duodenal drainage fluid after cholecystokinin (CCK) stimulation in healthy volunteers. Pancreas. 2002;**25**:350-354

[44] Suzuki T, Suzuki K, Kobayashi E, Ogawa Y, Kawamura Y, Nakai T, et al. Comparative study of the secretin test and pancreozymin secretin test in chronic pancreatitis. Nippon Shokakibyo Gakkai Zasshi. 1986;**83**:2209-2215

[45] Ceryak S, Steinberg WM, Marks ZH, Ruiz A. Feasibility of an endoscopic secretin test: Preliminary results. Pancreas. 2001;**23**:216-218

[46] et al. Slavova MK, Siminkovitch S, Gecov P, Genov J, Golemanov B, Mitova R, Up-to-date approach to monitor pancreatic exocrine insufficiency in adult patients with cystic fibrosis. International Journal of Medical Science

and Clinical invention. 2017;**4**(12):3358-3360. DOI: 10.18535/ijmsci/v4i12.06

[47] Bilgin M, Bilgin S, Balci NC, Momtahen AJ, Bilgin Y, Klör HU, et al. Magnetic resonance imaging and magnetic resonance cholangiopancreatography findings compared with fecal elastase 1 measurement for the diagnosis of chronic pancreatitis. Pancreas. 2008;**36**:e33-e39

[48] Sainani N et al. Evaluation of qualitative magnetic resonance imaging features for diagnosis of chronic pancreatitis. Pancreas. 2015;**44**:1280-1289

[49] Schneider AR, Hammerstingl R, Heller M, Povse N, Murzynski L, Vogl TJ, et al. Does secretin stimulated MRCP predict exocrine pancreatic insufficiency?: A comparison with noninvasive exocrine pancreatic function tests. Journal of Clinical Gastroenterology. 2006;**40**:851-855

[50] Trikudanathan G et al. Diagnostic performance of contrast-enhanced MRI with secretin-stimulated MRCP for non-calcific chronic pancreatitis: A comparison with histopathology. American Journal of Gastroenterology. 2015;**110**(11):1598-1606 (advance online publication)

[51] Tsai L and Lee K. Dynamic pancreatography with secretin-MRCP. Applied Radiology. 2015. pp. 34-38. Available from: www.appliedradiology

[52] Domínguez-Muñoz JE, Iglesias-García J, Vilariño-Insua M, Iglesias-Rey M. ^{13}C-mixed triglyceride breath test to assess oral enzyme substitution therapy in patients with chronic pancreatitis. Clinical Gastroenterology and Hepatology. 2007;**5**:484-488

[53] Bozek M, Jonderko K, Piłka M. On a refinement of the ^{13}C-mixed TAG breath test. The British Journal of Nutrition. 2012;**107**:211-217

[54] Iglesias-Garcia J, Vilarino M, Iglesias-Rey M, Lourido V, Dominguez-Munoz E. Accuracy of the optimized ^{13}C-mixed triglyceride breath test for the diagnosis of steatorrhea in clinical practice. Gastroenterology. 2003;**124**(Supp 1):A631

[55] Loser C, Brauer C, Aygen S, Hennemann O, Fölsch UR. Comparative clinical evaluation of the ^{13}C-mixed triglyceride breath test as an indirect pancreatic function test. Scandinavian Journal of Gastroenterology. 1998;**33**:327-334

[56] Vantrappen GR, Rutgeerts PJ, Ghoos YF, Hiele MI. Mixed triglyceride breath test: A noninvasive test of pancreatic lipase activity in the duodenum. Gastroenterology. 1989;**96**:1126-1134

[57] Scotta MS, Marzani MD, Maggiore G, De Giacomo C, Melzi D'Eril GV, Moratti R. Fecal chymotrypsin: A new diagnostic test for exocrine pancreatic insufficiency in children with cystic fibrosis. Clinical Biochemistry. 1985;**18**:233-234

[58] Bilgin M, Bilgin S, Balci NC, et al. Magnetic resonance imaging and magnetic resonance cholangiopancreatography findings compared with fecal elastase 1 measurement for the diagnosis of chronic pancreatitis. Pancreas. 2008;**36**:e33-e39

[59] Hardt PD, Marzeion AM, Schnell-Kretschmer H, Wüsten O, Nalop J, Zekorn T, et al. Fecal elastase 1 measurement compared with endoscopic retrograde cholangiopancreatography for the diagnosis of chronic pancreatitis. Pancreas. 2002;**25**:e6-e9

[60] Loser C, Möllgaard A, Fölsch UR. Faecal elastase 1: A novel, highly

sensitive, and specific tubeless pancreatic function test. Gut. 1996;**39**:580-586

[61] Pandol SJ. Neurohumoral control of exocrine pancreatic secretion. Current Opinion in Gastroenterology. 2003;**19**:443-446

[62] Sziegoleit A, Krause E, Klör HU, Kanacher L, Linder D. Elastase 1 and chymotrypsin B in pancreatic juice and feces. Clinical Biochemistry. 1989;**22**:85-89

[63] Fine KD, Ogunji F. A new method of quantitative fecal fat microscopy and its correlation with chemically measured fecal fat output. American Journal of Clinical Pathology. 2000;**113**:528-534

[64] Amann ST, Josephson SA, Toskes PP. Acid steatocrit: A simple, rapid gravimetric method to determine steatorrhea. The American Journal of Gastroenterology. 1997;**92**:2280-2284

[65] Sugai E, Srur G, Vazquez H, Benito F, Mauriño E, Boerr LA, et al. Steatocrit: A reliable semiquantitative method for detection of steatorrhea. Journal of Clinical Gastroenterology. 1994;**19**:206-209

[66] Van De Kamer JH, Ten Bokkel HH, Weyers HA. Rapid method for the determination of fat in feces. The Journal of Biological Chemistry. 1949;**177**:347-355

[67] Seiler CM, Izbicki J, Varga-Szabó L, Czakó L, Fiók J, Sperti C, et al. Randomised clinical trial: A 1-week, double-blind, placebocontrolled study of pancreatin 25 000 Ph. Eur. Minimicrospheres (Creon 25000 MMS) for pancreatic exocrine insufficiency after pancreatic surgery, with a 1-year open-label extension. Alimentary Pharmacology & Therapeutics. 2013;**37**:691-702

[68] Borowitz D et al. Coefficients of fat and nitrogen absorption in healthy subjects and individuals with cystic fibrosis. Journal of Pediatric Pharmacology and Therapeutics. 2007;**12**:47-52

[69] Darwin L et al. American pancreatic association practice guidelines in chronic pancreatitis. Pancreas. 2014;**43**(8):1143-1162

[70] Papazachariou IM, Martinez-Isla A, Efthimiou E, Williamson RC, Girgis SI. Magnesium deficiency in patients with chronic pancreatitis identified by an intravenous loading test. Clinica Chimica Acta. 2000;**302**:145-154

[71] Thorat V, Reddy N, Bhatia S, Bapaye A, Rajkumar JS, Kini DD, et al. Randomised clinical trial: The efficacy and safety of pancreatin enteric-coated minimicrospheres (Creon 40000 MMS) in patients with pancreatic exocrine insufficiency due to chronic pancreatitis—A double-blind, placebo-controlled study. Alimentary Pharmacology & Therapeutics. 2012;**36**:426-436

[72] Berry AJ. Pancreatic enzyme replacement therapy during pancreatic insufficiency. Nutrition in Clinical Practice. 2014;**29**:312-321. DOI: 10.1177/0884533614527773

[73] Dominguez-Munoz JE, Iglesias-Garcia J, Iglesias-Rey M, Figueiras A, Vilarino-Insua M. Effect of the administration schedule on the therapeutic efficacy of oral pancreatic enzyme supplements in patients with exocrine pancreatic insufficiency: A randomized, three-way crossover study. Alimentary Pharmacology & Therapeutics. 2005;**21**(8):993-1000

[74] Dominguez-Munoz JE, Iglesias-Garcia J, Iglesias-Rey M, et al. Effect of the administration schedule on the therapeutic efficacy of oral pancreatic enzyme supplements in patients with exocrine pancreatic insufficiency:

A randomized, three-way crossover study. Alimentary Pharmacology & Therapeutics. 2005;**21**:993-1000

[75] Ferrone M, Raimondo M, Scolapio JS. Pancreatic enzyme pharmacotherapy. Pharmacotherapy. 2007;**27**(6):910-920

[76] Fieker A, Philpott J. Armand M, Enzyme replacement therapy for pancreatic insufficiency: Present and future. Clinical and Experimental Gastroenterology. 2011;**4**:55-73

[77] Naikwade SR, Meshram RN, Bajaj AN. Preparation and in vivo efficacy study of pancreatin microparticles as an enzyme replacement therapy for pancreatitis. Drug Development and Industrial Pharmacy. 2009;**35**(4): 417-432

[78] Gubergrits N, Malecka-Panas E, Lehman GA, Vasileva G, Shen Y, Sander-Struckmeier S, et al. A 6-month, open-label clinical trial of pancrelipase delayed-release capsules (Creon) in patients with exocrine pancreatic insufficiency due to chronic pancreatitis or pancreatic surgery. Alimentary Pharmacology & Therapeutics. 2011;**33**:1152-1161

[79] Hoffmeister A et al. English language version of the S3-consensus guidelines on chronic pancreatitis: Definition, aetiology, diagnostic examinations, medical, endoscopic and surgical management of chronic pancreatitis. Gastroenterology. 2015;**53**:1447-1495

[80] Somaraju UR, Solis-Moya A. Pancreatic enzyme replacement therapy for people with cystic fibrosis. Cochrane Database of Systematic Reviews. 2014;**10**:CD008227

[81] Stern RC, Eisenberg JD, Wagener JS, et al. A comparison of the efficacy and tolerance of pancrelipase and placebo in the treatment of steatorrhea in cystic fibrosis patients with clinical

exocrine pancreatic insufficiency. The American Journal of Gastroenterology. 2000;**95**:1932-1938

[82] FitzSimmons SC, Burkhart GA, Borowitz D, Grand RJ, Hammerstrom T, Durie PR, et al. High-dose pancreatic-enzyme supplements and fibrosing colonopathy in children with cystic fibrosis. The New England Journal of Medicine. 1997;**336**:1283-1289. DOI: 10.1056/NEJM199705013361803

[83] Bruno MJ, Rauws EA, et al. Comparative effects of adjuvant cimetidine and omeprazole during pancreatic enzyme replacement therapy. Digestive Diseases and Sciences. 1994;**39**(5):988-992

[84] Decher N, Berry A. Post-whipple: A practical approach to nutrition management practical. Gastroenterology. 2012;**36**(8):30-42

[85] Keller J, Layer P. Human pancreatic exocrine response to nutrients in health and disease. Gut. 2005;**54**:1-28. DOI: 10.1136/gut.2005.065946

[86] Proesmans M, De Boeck K. Omeprazole, a proton pump inhibitor, improves residual steatorrhoea in cystic fibrosis patients treated with high dose pancreatic enzymes. European Journal of Pediatrics. 2003;**162**:760-763. DOI: 10.1007/s00431-003-1309-5

[87] Francisco MP, Wagner MH, Sherman JM, Theriaque D, Bowser E, Novak DA. Ranitidine and omeprazole as adjuvant therapy to pancrelipase to improve fat absorption in patients with cystic fibrosis. Journal of Pediatric Gastroenterology and Nutrition. 2002;**35**:79-83. DOI: 10.1097/00005176-200207000-00017

[88] Meier RF, Beglinger C. Nutrition in pancreatic diseases. Best Practice & Research Clinical Gastroenterology. 2006;**20**:507-529

[89] Meier R, Ockenga J, Pertkiewicz M, Pap A, Milinic N, Macfie J, et al. ESPEN guidelines on enteral nutrition: Pancreas. Clinical Nutrition. 2006;**25**:275-284

[90] Law R, Parsi M, Lopez R, Zuccaro G, Stevens T. Cigarette smoking is independently associated with chronic pancreatitis. Pancreatology. 2010;**10**:54-59. DOI: 10.1159/000225927

[91] Kovacheva-Slavova M, Siminkovitch S, Genov J, Golemanov B, Mitova R, Gecov P, et al. Nutritional deficiencies distribution in asymptomatic patients with pancreatic exocrine insufficiency due to chronic pancreatitis. 50 Annual Meeting of the European Pancreatic Club, Berlin, Germany, June 13-16, 2018. Pancreatology. 2018;**18**(4):S110

[92] Kovacheva-Slavova M, Siminkovitch S, Genov J, Golemanov B, Mitova R, Gecov P, et al. Monitoring and optimization of pancreatic enzyme replacement therapy in patients with pancreatic exocrine insufficiency. 25 United European Gastroenterology Week ; Barcelona Spain, October 28–November 01, 2017. United European Gastroenterology Journal. 2017;**5**(S1):A655

[93] Domínguez-Muñoz JE. Pancreatic enzyme replacement therapy for pancreatic exocrine insufficiency: When is it indicated, what is the goal and how to do it? Advances in Medical Sciences. 2011;**56**:1-5. DOI: 10.2478/v10039-011-0005-3

[94] Kovacheva-Slavova M, Siminkovitch S, Genov J, Golemanov B, Mitova R, Gecov P, et al. Pancreatic enzyme replacement therapy in patients with pancreatic exocrine insufficiency. Transylvanian Review. 2018;**XXVI**(24):6359-6362

[95] Kovacheva-Slavova M, Siminkovitch S, Genov J, Golemanov B, Mitova R, Gecov P, et al. Monitoring and optimization of pancreatic enzyme replacement therapy in patients with pancreatic exocrine insufficiency. 25 United European Gastroenterology Week; Barcelona Spain, October 28–November 01, 2017. United European Gastroenterology Journal. 2017;**5**(S1):A655

[96] Duggan SN, Smyth ND, Murphy A, Macnaughton D, O'Keefe SJ, Conlon KC. High prevalence of osteoporosis in patients with chronic pancreatitis: A systematic review and meta-analysis. Clinical Gastroenterology and Hepatology. 2014;**12**(2):219-228. DOI: 10.1016/j.cgh.2013.06.016 (Epub Jul 12, 2013)

[97] Haderslev KV, Jeppesen PB, Sorensen HA, Mortensen PB, Staun M. Vitamin D status and measurements of markers of bone metabolism in patients with small intestinal resection. Gut. 2003;**52**:653-658

[98] Hummel D, Aggarwal A, Borka K, Bajna E, Kállay E, Horváth HC. The vitamin D system is deregulated in pancreatic diseases. The Journal of Steroid Biochemistry and Molecular Biology. 2014;**144**:402-409. DOI: 10.1016/j.jsbmb.2014.07.011

[99] Czako L, Takacs T, Hegyi P, et al. Quality of life assessment after pancreatic enzyme replacement therapy in chronic pancreatitis. Canadian Journal of Gastroenterology. 2003;**17**:597-603

[100] Domínguez-Muñoz JE, Iglesias-García J. Oral pancreatic enzyme substitution therapy in chronic pancreatitis: Is clinical response an appropriate marker for evaluation of therapeutic efficacy? Journal of the Pancreas. 2010;**11**:158-162

[101] Somaraju UR, Solis-Moya A. Pancreatic enzyme replacement therapy for people with cystic fibrosis. Cochrane

Database of Systematic Reviews. 2014;**10**:CD008227

[102] Trang T, Chan J, Graham DY. Pancreatic enzyme replacement therapy for pancreatic exocrine insufficiency in the 21(st) century. World Journal of Gastroenterology. 2014;**20**:11467-11485. DOI: 10.3748/wjg. v20.i33.11467

[103] Siminkovitch S, Kovacheva-Slavova M, Vladimirov B, Genov J, Mitova R, Gecov P, et al. Evaluation of vitamin D, a, E status in patients with pancreatic disorders. 46 Annual Meeting of the American Pancreatic Association. San Diego California, November 4-7, 2015. Pancreas. 2015;**44**(8):1415-1416

[104] Kovacheva-Slavova M, Siminkovitch S, Vladimirov B, Genov J, Mitova R, Gecov P, et al. Relation between vitamin D status and cardiovascular risk factors in patients with chronic and recurrent pancreatitis—preliminary data. 24 United European Gastroenterology Week; Vienna, Austria, October 15-19, 2016. United European Gastroenterology Journal. 2016;**2**(S1):A187

[105] Bernstein CN, Leslie WD, Leboff MS. AGA technical review on osteoporosis in gastrointestinal diseases. Gastroenterology. 2003;**124**:795-841

[106] Mann ST, Stracke H, et al. Alterations of bone mineral density and bone metabolism in patients with various grades of chronic pancreatitis. Metabolism. 2003;**52**:579-585

[107] Maqbool A, Graham-Maar RC, et al. Vitamin A intake and elevated serum retinol levels in children and young adults with cystic fibrosis. Journal of Cystic Fibrosis. 2008;7:137-141

[108] Rovner A, Stallings V, Schall J, Leonard M, Zemel B. Vitamin D insufficiency in children, adolescents, and young adults with cystic fibrosis despite routine oral supplementation. American Journal of Clinical Nutrition. 2007;**86**:1694-1699

[109] Duggan SN, O'Sullivan M, Hamilton S, Feehan SM, Ridgway PF, Conlon KC. Patients with chronic pancreatitis are at increased risk for osteoporosis. Pancreas. 2012;**41**(7):1119-1124. DOI: 10.1097/ MPA.0b013e31824abb4d

[110] de la Iglesia-Garcia D, Vallejo-Senra N, Iglesias-Garcia J, López-López A, Nieto L, Domínguez-Muñoz JE. Increased risk of mortality associated with pancreatic exocrine insufficiency in patients with chronic pancreatitis. Journal of Clinical Gastroenterology. 2018;**52**(8):e63-e72. DOI: 10.1097/ MCG.0000000000000917

[111] Kovacheva-Slavova M, Siminkovitch S, Vladimirov B, Genov J, Mitova R, Gecov P, et al. Cardiovascular risk assessment in patients with chronic and recurrent pancreatitis—Preliminary data. 48 Annual Meeting of the European Pancreatic Club, Liverpool UK, July 06-09, 2016. Pancreatology. 2016;**16**(3S1):S16

[112] Kaneva AM, Potolitsyna NN, Bojko ER, Odland JØ. The apolipoprotein B/ apolipoprotein A-I ratio as a potential marker of plasma atherogenicity. Disease Markers. 2015;**2015**:591454. DOI: 10.1155/2015/591454

[113] Kovacheva-Slavova M, Siminkovitch S, Genov J, Mitova R, Golemanov B, Gecov P, et al. Overall cardiovascular risk assessment in patients with chronic pancreatitis and exocrine insufficiency receiving enzyme replacement therapy. 26 United European Gastroenterology Week ; Vienna Austria, October 20-24, 2018. United European Gastroenterology Journal. 2018;**6**(S1):A655

[114] European Association for Cardiovascular Prevention & Rehabilitation et al. ESC/EAS guidelines for the management of dyslipidaemias: The task force for the management of dyslipidaemias of the European Society of Cardiology (ESC) and the European Atherosclerosis Society (EAS). European Heart Journal. 2011;**32**(14):1769-1818

[115] National Vascular Disease Prevention Alliance. Guidelines for the Management of Absolute Cardiovascular Disease Risk. 2012

[116] Anderson TJ et al. 2012 update of the Canadian Cardiovascular Society guidelines for the diagnosis and treatment of dyslipidemia for the prevention of cardiovascular disease in the adult. The Canadian Journal of Cardiology. 2013 Feb;**29**(2):151-167

[117] Goff DC Jr et al. 2013 ACC/AHA guideline on the assessment of cardiovascular risk: A report of the American College of Cardiology/American Heart Association Task Force on Practice Guidelines. Circulation. 2014;**129**(25 Suppl 2):S49-S73. DOI: 10.1161/01.cir.0000437741.48606.98 (Epub Nov 12, 2013)

[118] Boekholdt SM, Arsenault BJ, Mora S, et al. Association of LDL cholesterol, non-HDL cholesterol, and apolipoprotein B levels with risk of cardiovascular events among patients treated with statins: A meta-analysis. Journal of the American Medical Association. 2012;**307**:1302-1309

[119] Steffen BT, Guan W, Remaley AT, et al. Use of lipoprotein particle measures for assessing coronary heart disease risk post-American Heart Association/American College of Cardiology guidelines: The multi-ethnic study of atherosclerosis. Arteriosclerosis, Thrombosis, and Vascular Biology. 2015;**35**(2):448-454

[120] Sniderman AD, Williams K, Contois JH, et al. A meta-analysis of low density lipoprotein cholesterol, non-high-density lipoprotein cholesterol, and apolipoprotein B as markers of cardiovascular risk. Circulation. Cardiovascular Quality and Outcomes. 2011;**4**:337-345

[121] Contois JH, McConnell JP, Sethi AA, et al. Apolipoprotein B and cardiovascular disease risk: Position statement from the AACC lipoproteins and vascular diseases division working group on best practices. Clinical Chemistry. 2009;**55**(3):407-419

[122] Creutzfeldt W, Gleichmann D, Otto J, et al. Follow-up of exocrine pancreatic function in type-1 diabetes mellitus. Digestion. 2005;**72**(2-3):71-75

[123] Third Report of the National Cholesterol Education Program (NCEP) Expert Panel on Detection, Evaluation, and Treatment of High Blood Cholesterol in Adults (Adult Treatment Panel III) Final Report NIH Publication No. 02-5215 September 2002

[124] Thompson A, Danesh J. Associations between apolipoprotein B, apolipoprotein AI, the apolipoprotein B/AI ratio and coronary heart disease: A literature-based meta-analysis of prospective studies. Journal of Internal Medicine. 2006;**259**(5):481-492

[125] Andrikoula M, McDowell IFW. The contribution of ApoB and ApoA1 measurements to cardiovascular risk assessment diabetes. Obesity and Metabolism. 2008;**10**:271-278

[126] Kaneva A, Potolitsyna N, Bojko E, Odland J. The apolipoprotein B/apolipoprotein A-I ratio as a potential marker of plasma atherogenicity. Disease Markers. 2015;**2015**:7 p. Article ID: 591454

[127] Walldius G. The apoB/apoA-I ratio is a strong predictor of cardiovascular

risk. In: Frank S, Kostner G, editors. Lipoproteins in Health and Diseases. Rijeka, Croatia: InTech; 2012. pp. 95-148

[128] Schianca GPC, Pedrazzoli R, Onolfo S, et al. ApoB/apoA-I ratio is better than LDL-C in detecting cardiovascular risk. Nutrition, Metabolism and Cardiovascular Diseases. 2011;**21**(6):406-411. DOI: 10.1016/j.numecd.2009.11.002

[129] Yusuf S, Hawken S, Ounpuu S, et al. Effect of potentially modifiable risk factors associated with myocardial infarction in 52 countries (the INTERHEART study): Case-control study. The Lancet. 2004;**364**(9438):937-952

[130] Walldius G. Jungner I, Apolipoprotein B and apolipoprotein A-I: risk indicators of coronary heart disease and targets for lipid-modifying therapy. Journal of Internal Medicine. 2004;**255**:188-205

[131] Schmidt C, Fagerberg B, Wikstrand J, Hulthe J. ApoB/apoA-I ratio is related to femoral artery plaques and is predictive for future cardiovascular events in healthy men. Atherosclerosis. 2006;**189**(1):178-185. DOI: 10.1016/j. atherosclerosis.2005.11.031

[132] Marcovina S, Packard CJ. Measurement and meaning of apolipoprotein AI and apolipoprotein B plasma levels. Journal of Internal Medicine. 2006;**259**(5):437-446. DOI: 10.1111/j.1365-2796.2006.01648.x

[133] Lima LM, Carvalho MG, Sousa M. O, Apo B/apo A-I ratio and cardiovascular risk prediction. Arquivos Brasileiros de Cardiologia. 2007;**88**(6):e140-e143

[134] Ginsberg HN, Brown VW. Apolipoprotein C III. Arteriosclerosis, Thrombosis, and Vascular Biology. 2011;**31**:471-473

[135] Kovacheva-Slavova M, Siminkovitch S, Genov J, Mitova R, Gecov P, Golemanov B, et al. Apolipoproteins A-I, A-II, B, C-III as cardiovascular risk factors in patients with pancreatic disorders. 49 Annual Meeting of the European Pancreatic Club. Budapest Hungary, June 28–July 1, 2017. Pancreatology. 2017;**17**(3S):S108

[136] Lee SJ, Campos H, Moye LA, Sacks FM. LDL containing apolipoprotein CIII is an independent risk factor for coronary events in diabetic patients. Arteriosclerosis, Thrombosis, and Vascular Biology. 2003 May 1;**23**(5):853-858 (Epub Mar 13, 2003)

[137] Taskinen MR, Borén J. Why is apolipoprotein CIII emerging as a novel therapeutic target to reduce the burden of cardiovascular disease? Current Atherosclerosis Reports. 2016;**18**:59. DOI: 10.1007/s11883-016-0614-1

[138] Ewald N, Kaufmann C, Raspe A, et al. Prevalence of diabetes mellitus secondary to pancreatic diseases (type 3c). Diabetes/Metabolism Research and Reviews. 2012;**28**:338-342

[139] Hardt PD, Brendel MD, Kloer HU, Bretzel RG. Is pancreatic diabetes (type 3c diabetes) underdiagnosed and misdiagnosed? Diabetes Care. 2008;**31**(Suppl 2):S165-S169

[140] Rickels MR et al. Detection, evaluation and treatment of diabetes mellitus in chronic pancreatitis: Recommendations from PancreasFest 2012. Pancreatology. 2013;**13**:336-342

[141] Piciucchi M, Capurso G, Archibugi L, Delle Fave MM, Capasso M, Delle FG. Exocrine pancreatic insufficiency in diabetic patients: Prevalence, mechanisms, and treatment. International Journal of Endocrinology. 2015;**2015**:595649. DOI: 10.1155/2015/595649

[142] Riddle MC, American diabetes association standards of medical care in diabetes. The Journal of Clinical and Applied Research and Education. 2018;**41**(Supplement 1);S1-S159. ISSN: 0149-5992

[143] Kovacheva-Slavova M, Mitova-Siminkovitch S, Vladimirov B, Genov J, Gecov P, Mitova R. Diabetes mellitus type 3c screening by patients with chronic pancreatitis. 47 Annual Meeting of the European Pancreatic Club, Toledo Spain, June 24-26, 2015. Pancreatology. 2015;**15**(3S):S75

[144] Dhar P, Kalghatgi S, Saraf V. Pancreatic cancer in chronic pancreatitis. Indian Journal of Surgical Oncology. 2015;**6**(1):57-62

[145] Kong X, Sun T, Kong F, Du Y, Li Z. Chronic pancreatitis and pancreatic cancer. Gastrointest Tumors. 2014;**1**(3):123-134

[146] Augustine P, Ramesh H. Is tropical pancreatitis premalignant? The American Journal of Gastroenterology. 1992;**87**(8):1005-1008

[147] Mayerle J, Kalthoff H, et al Metabolic biomarker signature to differentiate pancreatic ductal adenocarcinoma from chronic pancreatitis. Gut. 2018;**67**:128-137

[148] Ramsey ML, Conwell DL, Hart PA. Complications of chronic pancreatitis. Digestive Diseases and Sciences. 2017;**62**(7):1745-1750. DOI: 10.1007/s10620-017-4518-x

[149] Hao L et al. Incidence of and risk factors for pancreatic cancer in chronic pancreatitis: A cohort of 1656 patients. Digestive and Liver Disease. 2017;**49**(11):1249-1256

[150] Barthet M, Bugallo M, Moreira LS, et al. Management of cysts and pseudocysts complicating chronic pancreatitis. A retrospective study of 143 patients. Gastroentérologie Clinique et Biologique. 1993;**17**:270-276

[151] Lerch MM, Stier A, Wahnschaffe U, et al. Pancreatic pseudocysts: Observation, endoscopic drainage, or resection? Deutsches Ärzteblatt International. 2009;**106**:614-621

[152] Jacobson BC, Baron TH, Adler DG, et al. ASGE guideline: The role of endoscopy in the diagnosis and the management of cystic lesions and inflammatory fluid collections of the pancreas. Gastrointestinal Endoscopy. 2005;**61**:363-370

[153] Samuelson AL, Shah RJ. Endoscopic management of pancreatic pseudocysts. Gastroenterology Clinics of North America. 2012;**41**:47-62

[154] Barthet M, Lamblin G, Gasmi M, et al. Clinical usefulness of a treatment algorithm for pancreatic pseudocysts. Gastrointestinal Endoscopy. 2008;**67**:245-252

[155] Gouyon B, Lévy P, Ruszniewski P, et al. Predictive factors in the outcome of pseudocysts complicating alcoholic chronic pancreatitis. Gut. 1997;**41**:821-825

[156] Lankisch PG, Weber-Dany B, Maisonneuve P, et al. Pancreatic pseudocysts: Prognostic factors for their development and their spontaneous resolution in the setting of acute pancreatitis. Pancreatology. 2012;**12**:85-90

[157] Butler JR, Eckert GJ, Zyromski NJ, Leonardi MJ, Lillemoe KD, Howard TJ. Natural history of pancreatitis-induced splenic vein thrombosis: A systematic review and meta-analysis of its incidence and rate of gastrointestinal bleeding. HPB: The

Official Journal of the International Hepato Pancreato Biliary Association. 2011;**13**(12):839-845

[158] Sakorafas GH, Sarr MG, Farley DR, Farnell MB. The significance of sinistral portal hypertension complicating chronic pancreatitis. American Journal of Surgery. 2000;**179**(2):129-133

[159] Weber SM, Rikkers LF. Splenic vein thrombosis and gastrointestinal bleeding in chronic pancreatitis. World Journal of Surgery. 2003;**27**(11):1271-1274 (Epub Oct 13, 2003)

[160] Simpson WG, Schwartz RW, Strodel WE. Splenic vein thrombosis. Southern Medical Journal. 1990;**83**(4):417-421

[161] Agarwal AK, Raj Kumar K, Agarwal S, et al. Significance of splenic vein thrombosis in chronic pancreatitis. American Journal of Surgery. 2008;**196**:149-154

[162] Levy MJ, Wong Kee Song LM. EUS-guided angiotherapy for gastric varices: Coil, glue, and sticky issues. Gastrointestinal Endoscopy. 2013;**78**:722-725

[163] DeSouza K, Nodit L. Groove pancreatitis: A brief review of a diagnostic challenge. Archives of Pathology & Laboratory Medicine. 2015;**139**(3):417-421. DOI: 10.5858/arpa.2013-0597-RS

[164] Vijungco J, Prinz R. Management of biliary and duodenal complications of chronic pancreatitis. World Journal of Surgery. 2003;**27**:1258-1270

[165] Adsay NV, Zamboni G. Paraduodenal pancreatitis: A clinico-pathologically distinct entity unifying "cystic dystrophy of heterotopic pancreas", "Para-duodenal wall cyst", and "groove pancreatitis". Seminars in Diagnostic Pathology. 2004;**21**(4):247-254

[166] Arora A et al. Paraduodenal pancreatitis. Clinical Radiology. 2014;**69**(3):299-306

[167] Díaz-Jaime FC, Herreras-Lopez J, et al. Groove pancreatitis: A description of four cases and literature review. International Journal of Digestive Diseases. 2016;**2**:1. DOI: 10.4172/2472-1891.100012

[168] Arora A, Rajesh S, Mukund A, et al. Clinicoradiological appraisal of 'paraduodenal pancreatitis': Pancreatitis outside the pancreas! The Indian Journal of Radiology & Imaging. 2015;**25**(3):303-314

[169] Egorov V, Vankovich A, Petrov R, et al., Pancreas-preserving approach to "Paraduodenal Pancreatitis" treatment: Why, when, and how? experience of treatment of 62 patients with duodenal dystrophy," BioMed Research International, 2014;**2014**:17 p. Article ID 185265

[170] Carvalho D, Loureiro R, Pavão Borges V, Russo P, Bernardes C, Ramos G. Paraduodenal pancreatitis: Three cases with different therapeutic approaches. GE Portuguese Journal of Gastroenterology. 2016;**24**(2):89-94

[171] Saluja SS, Kalayarasan R, Mishra PK, Srivastava S, Chandrasekar S, Godhi S. Chronic pancreatitis with benign biliary obstruction: Management issues. World Journal of Surgery. 2014;**38**(9):2455-2459. DOI: 10.1007/s00268-014-2581-4

[172] Aranha GV, Prinz RA, Freeark RJ, Greenlee HB. The spectrum of biliary tract obstruction from chronic pancreatitis. Archives of Surgery. 1984;**119**(5):595-600. DOI: 10.1001/archsurg.1984.01390170091018

[173] Abdallah AA, Krige JE, Bornman PC. Biliary tract obstruction in chronic pancreatitis. HPB: The Official Journal

of the International Hepato Pancreato
Biliary Association. 2007;**9**(6):421-428

[174] Hsu JT, Yeh CN, Hung CF,
Chen HM, Hwang TL, Jan YY,
et al. Management and outcome of
bleeding pseudoaneurysm associated
with chronic pancreatitis. BMC
Gastroenterology. 2006;**6**:3. DOI:
10.1186/1471-230X-6-3

[175] Mathew G, Bhimji SS. Pancreatic
pseudoaneurysm [Updated Nov 14,
2018]. In: StatPearls [Internet]. Treasure
Island (FL): StatPearls Publishing; 2018.
Available from: https://www.ncbi.nlm.
nih.gov/books/NBK430937/

[176] Mathew G, Bhimji SS. Aneurysm,
Pancreatic Pseudoaneurysm. Treasure
Island, FL: StatPearls Publishing; 2017

[177] Harvey J et al. Endovascular
management of hepatic artery
pseudoaneurysm hemorrhage
complicating pancreaticoduodenectomy.
Journal of Vascular Surgery.
2006;**43**(3):613-617

[178] Bender JS, Levison MA. Massive
hemorrhage associated with pancreatic
pseudocyst: Successful treatment
by pancreaticoduodenectomy. The
American Surgeon. 1991;**57**(10):653-655

[179] Jain G, Kathuria S, Nigam A,
Trehan VK. Transcatheter embolization
of a giant pancreatic pseudoaneurysm:
A tale of two bleeds and one thrombus!
Indian Heart Journal. 2013;**65**(1):91-94

[180] Choi EK, Lehman GA. Update
on endoscopic management of main
pancreatic duct stones in chronic calcific
pancreatitis. The Korean Journal of
Internal Medicine. 2012;**27**(1):20-29

[181] Vladimirov B, Getzov P, Ivanova R.
Endoscopic treatment of pancreatic
diseases. In: Amornyotin Somchai
editor. Endoscopy. IntechOpen 24 sept
2015. DOI: 10.5772/60589

[182] Correia M, Amonkar D, Audi P,
Banswal L, Samant D. Pancreatic calculi:
A case report and review of literature.
Saudi Surgical Journal. 2013;**1**:14-18

[183] Tandan M, Talukdar R, Reddy
DN. Management of pancreatic
calculi: An update. Gut Liver.
2016;**10**(6):873-880

[184] Aaronson NK, Ahmedzai S,
Bergman B, Bullinger M, Cull A, Duez
NJ, et al. The European Organization
for Research and Treatment of
cancer QLQ-C30: A quality-of-life
instrument for use in international
clinical trials in oncology. Journal
of the National Cancer Institute.
1993;**85**(5):365-376

[185] Fitzsimmons D, Kahl S, Butturini G,
et al. Symptoms and quality of life
in chronic pancreatitis assessed by
structured interview and the EORTC
QLQC30 and QLQ-PAN26. The
American Journal of Gastroenterology.
2005;**100**:918-926

[186] Mokrowiecka A, Pinkowski D,
Malecka-Panas E, Johnson CD.
Clinical, emotional and social
factors associated with quality
of life in chronic pancreatitis.
Pancreatology. 2010;**10**(1):39-46. DOI:
10.1159/000225920 (Epub Mar 20,
2010)

[187] JanChrastina J, Bednářová D,
Ludíková L. Quality of life in
patients with chronic pancreatitis—
Possibilities of measurement of the
phenomenon in research. Kontakt. June
2015;**17**(2):e89-e95

[188] Lee V, Cheng H, Li G, Saif MW.
Quality of life in patients with
pancreatic cancer. Journal of the
Pancreas: JOP. 2012;**13**(2):182-184

[189] Machicado JD, Amann ST,
Anderson MA, Abberbock J, Sherman S,
Conwell DL, et al. Quality of life in
chronic pancreatitis is determined

by constant pain, disability/
unemployment, current smoking,
and associated co-morbidities. The
American Journal of Gastroenterology.
2017;**112**(4):633-642

[190] Balliet WB, Edwards-Hampton S,
Borckardt JJ, et al. Depressive
symptoms, pain, and quality of life
among patients with nonalcohol-related
chronic pancreatitis. Pain Research and
Treatment. 2012;**2012**:5 p. Article ID
978646. DOI: 10.1155/2012/978646

Chapter 5

Pediatric Pancreatitis: Not a Rare Entity

Stefano Valabrega, Laura Bersigotti, Laura Antolino,

Paolo Aurello, Federico Tomassini, P. Valabrega, S. Amato,

Francesco D'Angelo, Luciano Izzo and Salvatore Caterino

Abstract

The incidence of acute pancreatitis is increasing in children and it should be considered as part of differential diagnosis in case of abdominal pain. The etiology of acute pancreatitis in this subpopulation is related to several conditions and risk factors, such as drugs, obesity, infections, trauma and anatomic abnormalities. In older children abdominal pain is the first symptom in more than 90% of cases, where as in younger children vomiting represents an early clinical manifestation. Diagnosis is based on laboratory investigation, such as serum levels of lipase, and imaging findings (ultrasonography, CT scanning or MRI) such as detecting edema, hemorrage or necrosis of pancreatic parenchyma or in peripancreatic fat. Treatments for adults and children are similar. Rapid and accurate assessment of the severity of pancreatitis is absolutely indicated for selecting the appropriate treatment and predicting the prognosis.

Keywords: pancreatitis, children, abdominal pain, severity assessment

1. Introduction

Pediatric pancreatitis has increased in incidence during last decades and 1/10,000 children per year is affected by the acute form genetic mutations and congenital abnormalities represent the major risk factors for this disease but there is no agreement about a certain pathogenetic theory. The reasons of pancreatitis' burden in pediatric population may be multifactorial and it can be explained by an improved detection instead of a real increase [1].

In children, pancreatitis is categorized as acute pancreatitis (AP), acute recurrent pancreatitis (ARP) and chronic pancreatitis (CP). Here we summarize recent advances in the field of pediatric pancreatitis with focus on etiologies, pathogenesis, diagnosis and therapy.

2. Acute pancreatitis

Acute pancreatitis (AP), in children is increasingly recognized to be a challenge for affected patients and their families, their treating physicians and surgeons, and the health care system. The incidence of pediatric AP was estimated at 3.6–13.2 per

100,000 per children per year, which is within of the range of incidence reported for adult AP. Genetic contributions to the development of pancreatitis, especially in acute recurrent and chronic pancreatitis are now increasingly recognized. There are no evidence-based diagnostic guidelines for pancreatic disorders in children. The diagnosis criteria are based on symptoms, biochemical and imaging evidence of pancreatitis, with two of the three criteria required to diagnose AP. A multicenter effort led by INSPPIRE (INternational Study Group of Pediatric Pancreatitis: In Search for a CuRE) defined AP as requiring 2 of: (1) abdominal pain compatible with AP, (2) serum amylase and/or lipase values ≥3 times upper limits of normal, (3) imaging findings consistent with AP. Although abdominal pain is the most common clinical manifestation, it may be absent in up to one third of pediatric patients. The diagnostic yield and concordances for serum pancreatic enzymes and imaging for the diagnosis of pediatric AP will be discusses. Pediatric AP is associated with significant disease burden. There is currently no consensus on the definition for severity of AP in children. However, there are now predictors of severity for AP that has been developed and validated in children. The management of AP remains driven by adult studies and recommendations. Treatment is directed at the underlying etiologies as well as supportive measures.

2.1 Etiology

While alcohol and gallstones represent the main causes of acute pancreatitis in adult population, the etiological scenario of acute pancreatitis is mostly due to drugs, infectious diseases, congenital abnormalities or trauma (**Table 1**). Furthermore etiological factors may vary considerably according with ethnicity.

2.1.1 Infections

Pediatric acute pancreatitis is associated with paramyxovirus or mycoplasma infections. Mumps virus induces parotitis and orchitis in pediatric population and may be complicated by meningoencephalitis or pancreatitis. In the latter case clinical manifestations are represented by usually self-limiting diarrhea and abdominal pain. Mycoplasma infection-related pancreatitis can be distinguished into two types: early onset type and late-onset type following respiratory tract symptoms beginning. This different onset spectrum is due to a direct injury of mycoplasma into the acinar cells in the former type while to an autoantibodies targeting in the latter [2].

2.1.2 Congenital abnormalities

Chole-dochal cyst constitutes the most principal cause of AP. In case of abnormal junction between pancreatic and biliary ducts the sphincter of Oddi encircles

Common	Less common	Rare
Biliary disorders	Infections	Autoimmune pancreatitis
Systemic conditions	Metabolic diseases	Anatomic pancreatobiliary abnormalities
Medications	Genetic/hereditary	
Trauma		
Idiopathic		

Table 1.
Causes of acute pancreatitis in children.

a single channel leading to bile reflux into the Wirsung duct is communication between in course of sphincter contraction or bilestone impingement in the common channel [3].

2.1.3 Drugs and chemotherapeutic agents

Drug-induced acute pancreatitis accounts for 21% of all cases in pediatric population. Valproic acid, radiocontrast and corticosteroids can induce pancreatitis in the context of epilepsy or inflammatory bowel diseases [4].

L-asparaginase-associated pancreatitis (AAP) occurs in 0.7–24% of children treated for acute lymphoblastic leukemia with mortality rates of 2–5%. Older children demonstrate an high risk for developing acute pancreatitis and if it occurs they could experience cancer recurrence [5].

2.1.4 Trauma

Pediatric pancreatic injuries are uncommon and can be mostly ascribed to vehicle accidents. Anyway because of its retroperitoneal location pancreas is preserved in case of minor abdominal traumas and a pancreatic transection can occur clinically silent [6].

2.2 Pathophysiology

Acute pancreatitis is due to an organ injury with a subsequent inflammatory response that may involve both adjacent and distant structures. The first pathogenetic event may be represented by an acinar cell injury (**Figure 1**) that produces pancreatic edema with the activation of the inflammatory pathway. The release of cytokines and chemokines leads to a systemic inflammatory response (SIRS) and to complications such as pancreatic necrosis, shock and distant organ failure.

Several hypotheses have been advanced explaining the mechanism of this acinar cell damage. The autodigestion model focused on a premature calcium-mediated intracellular trypsinogen activation in trypsin (**Figure 1**). Trypsin then activates digestive enzymes that mediate acinar cell injury. On the other hand, recent studies in animal models of AP highlight the pathogenetic role of colocalized zymogens and lysosomes, intra acinar activation of zymogens, nuclear factor-κb activation and inhibition of secretion [7].

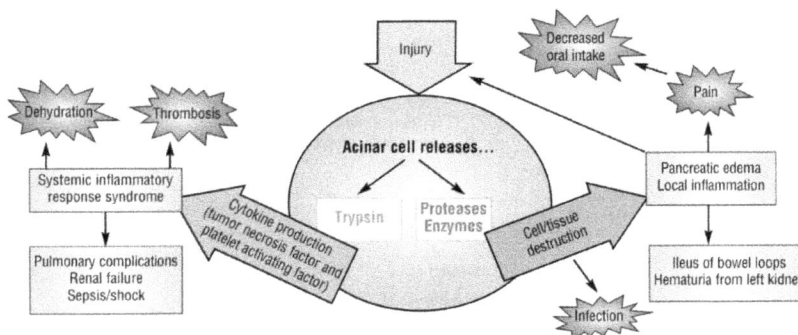

Figure 1.
Pathophysiology of acute pancreatitis.

2.3 Diagnosis

The diagnosis of AP in children depends on clinical manifestations, laboratory tests, and imaging. Moreover a careful estimation of severity is fundamental for establish the most appropriate treatment (**Figure 2**).

2.3.1 Clinical features

There are differences in clinical onset and natural course between adults and children. Acute pancreatitis symptoms are non-specific and depend on child's age and developmental level. Abdominal pain is typically epigastric but it can be localized to the right upper quadrant or left upper one. It can occur constantly or intermittently, with radiation to the back. The pain is dull, boring and deep. Pancreatitis should be suspected in all pediatric patients who experience, as isolated or combined symptoms, abdominal pain, nausea and/or vomit, the latter due to peripancreatic inflammation extended to the gastric wall [8].

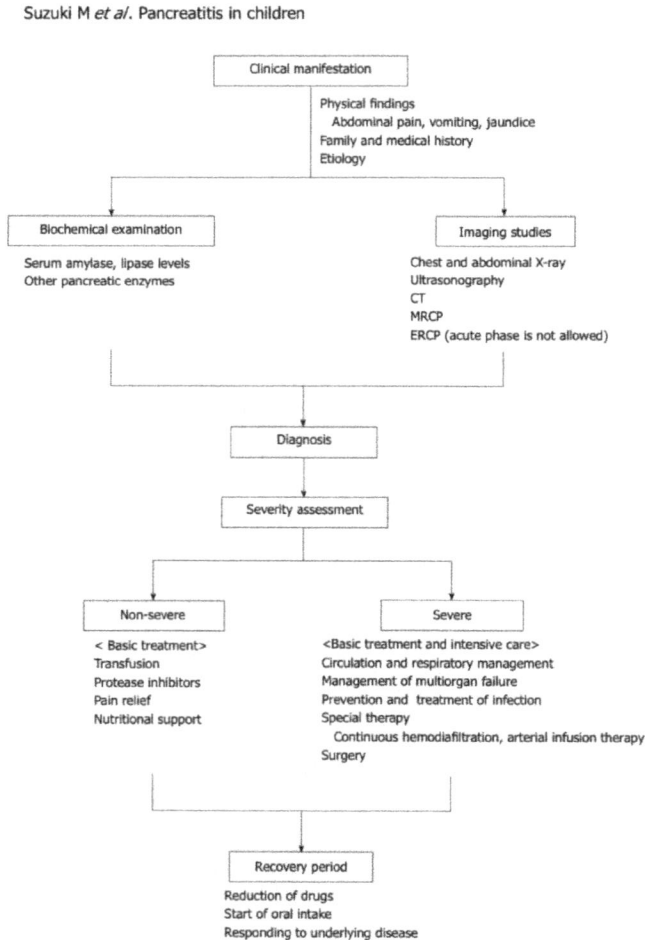

Figure 2.
Pediatric acute pancreatitis diagnostic flow chart.

2.3.2 Biochemical tests

The increased serum levels of amylase enzyme greater than three upper limits of normal are also detected in case of pancreatobiliary tract obstruction and perforative peritonitis, in addition to salivary gland pathologies and renal failure. Therefore this parameter is associated with a low specificity. On the other hand serum lipase levels have a sensitivity of 86.5–100% and specificity of 84.7–99.0%. In case of severe pancreatitis, serum lipase levels seven times higher than normal have been detected within the first 24 h. It is important to underline that in case of drug-induced acute pancreatitis serum amylase may not be elevate [9]. In addition, we may consider other chemistry panels to define a diagnosis like serum calcium, electrolytes, urea nitrogen, creatinine, transaminases, albumin, bilirubin, triglycerides and blood cell count [10].

2.3.3 Diagnostic imaging

Transabdominal ultrasound is the diagnostic study of choice to evaluate biliary tree abnormalities in children. In pediatric age pancreatic head tend to be larger than body and tail and this is a potentially confounding feature that may lead to a misdiagnosis. Diffuse or focal enlargement of the pancreatic gland may be present in AP and is attributable to edema. Echogenicity is a variable feature in case of pediatric pancreatitis, however hypoechogenicity is frequently seen.

One of the most valid radiological finding is represented by the dilatation of the pancreatic duct (1–6 years old, >1.5 mm; 7–12 years old, >1.9 mm; 13–18 years, >2.2 mm). Poorly defined borders or localized intraparenchymal fluid collection are usually detected at ultrasound imaging in the acute setting.

Parenchymal hypodensities, heterogeneity, irregularity of the glandular margins and inflammatory changes in the peripancreatic fat could be seen at CT (computed tomography) scans. The use of intravenous contrast is mandatory to evaluate different grades of glandular involvement and patency of adjacent vessels. Furthermore, CT imaging may show the extent of peripancreatic or intraparenchymal fluid collections and the presence abscessualization.

Magnetic resonance cholangiopancreatography (MRCP) is challenging o perform in pediatric patients and needs to be tailored to different body sizes. The pancreatic glands become heterogeneous and hypointense on T1-weighted images in the early stages of inflammation [11].

2.3.4 Severity assessment

Commonly used scoring systems (Ranson, modified Glasgow and pediatric acute pancreatitis severity) have demonstrated limited ability to predict disease severity in children and adolescents with acute pancreatitis. The sensitivity and negative predictive value of the above scores are insufficient to guide decision making in pediatric patients. Therefore better methods are needed for risk stratification. Anyway, in a logistic regression model [12], only white blood cell count at admission more than 18,500/mcL, trough calcium less than 8.3 mg/dL and blood urea nitrogen greater than 5 mg/dL appear to correspond independently with a poor outcome.

The lack of an accurate scoring system could cause delays in appropriate clinical management and increase the risk of progressive life-threatening complications. In recent years Suzuki [13] has investigated a modified score that reflects pediatric SIRS (systemic inflammatory response syndrome) score, age and weight (**Figure 3**) and it has proved a more adequate scoring system in children, helping to improve treatment outcome in these patients.

Parameter	Pediatric JPN scoring system[a]
1	Base excess < -3 mEq or shock
2	$PaO_2 < 60$ mmHg in room air or respiratory failure requiring ventilation
3	BUN > 40 mg/dl or creatinine >2 mg/dl or urine output <0.5 ml/kg/h
4	LDH > 2 times above the upper limit of normal (age adjusted values)
5	Platelet count $< 1,00,000$ cells/cu.mm
6	Total serum calcium <7.5 mg/dl
7	C-reactive protein > 15 mg/dl
8	Number of positive measures in pediatric SIRS score > 3 [SIRS criteria A: Core temperature > 38.53 °C or <36 °C B. Tachycardia– mean heart rate >2SD above normal for age C. Tachypnea– mean respiratory rate >2SD above normal for age D. Leucocyte count either elevated or depressed for age or >10 % immature neutrophils]
9	Age less than 7 y and/or weight below 23 kg

[a] Presence of any three of the above criteria indicates severe pancreatitis

Figure 3.
Japanese scoring system to assess severity of acute pancreatitis.

2.3.5 Complications

The most frequent complication of acute pancreatitis in pediatric age is represented by the development of pseudocysts and occurs in 13% of patients (**Figure 4**). This is a delayed complication and occurs 4 weeks after the onset of the acute inflammatory process. Pseudocysts probably arise from disruption of the main pancreatic duct, leading to an oval fluid collection with a well-defined wall in the peripancreatic tissues. The early alteration that involves pancreatic tissue in the setting of an interstitial edematous pancreatitis (IEP) is the formation of peripancreatic fluid collections that may resolve spontaneously. A necrotizing process arising in the pancreatic parenchyma or in adjacent tissues results in the development of multiple necrotic collections walled-off with an increased risk of infection.

Vascular complications may involve the arterial or venous system and are caused by extravasated pancreatic enzymes with the loss of vessel wall integrity. Thus hemorrhage secondary to the rupture of a pseudoaneurysm or erosion of a major artery may occur. Moreover, in the venous system, thrombosis is a complication that commonly affects the splenic vein. Pancreatic ascites and pancreaticopleural fistulas are two uncommon types of internal pancreatic fistulas resulting from pancreatic duct disruption with leakage of pancreatic fluid. Since complications are similar to those occurring in adults the revised Atlanta classification (**Figure 5**) is useful in children too [11].

Intra-abdominal hypertension (IAH) and abdominal compartment syndrome (ACS) are rare in children with severe acute pancreatitis but still have high mortality rates.

The increased abdominal pressure leads to alteration in microvasculature determining ischemia, congestion and edema of the organs. Thus the consequent

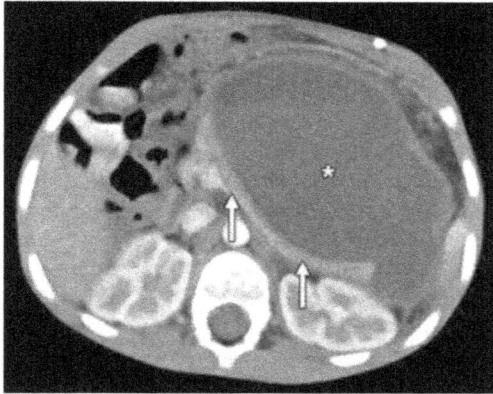

Figure 4.
Pancreatic pseudocyst at contrast-enhanced CT scan in a 6-year old patient.

Type of Pancreatitis   Fluid Collections

< 4 Weeks after Onset

IEP   APFC
          Sterile
          Infected

Necrotizing Pancreatitis   ANC
          Parencymal necrosis alone
          Sterile
          Infected
          Peripancreatic necrosis alone
          Sterile
          Infected
          Pancreatic and peripancreatic necrosis
          Sterile
          Infected

≥ 4 Weeks after Onset

IEP   Pancreatic pseudocyst
          Sterile
          Infected

Necrotizing Pancreatitis   WON
          Sterile
          Infected

Figure 5.
Revised Atlanta classification of complications in AP. IEP: interstitial edematous pancreatitis; APFC: acute peripancreatic fluid collection; ANC: acute necrotic collection; WON: walled-off necrosis.

bacterial shift into the bloodstream causes bacteremia, systemic inflammatory response and hemodynamic instability. The purpose of management of critical pediatric patients is to avoid ACS progression and the development of multi-organ dysfunction syndrome [14].

2.4 Treatment

2.4.1 Drug therapy

Children with AP should be resuscitated with crystalloids and be provided 1.5–2 times maintenance intravenous fluids with monitoring of urine output over the next 24–48 h. Monitoring of patients with acute pancreatitis can provide indicators of complications arising, including SIRS and organ dysfunction/failure. Cardiac, respiratory, and renal status should be followed particularly closely within the first 48 h. Opioid analgesics in oral or parenteral forms are required for pain control in acute pancreatitis. Despite previous contentions, there is no evidence about the paradoxical contraction of the sphincter of Oddi induced by morphin and it should be used for acute pancreatitis pain not responding to acetaminophen or NSAIDs (non steroids anti-inflammatory drugs). In pediatric patients with a diagnosis of mild acute pancreatitis oral feedings or enteral nutrition (EN) can be started within 24–48 h. Parenteral nutrition (PN) should be considered in cases where EN is not possible for a prolonged period (longer than 5–7 days) such as in ileus, complex fistulae, abdominal compartment syndrome, to reduce the catabolic state of the body.

Antibiotics should not be used in the management of AP, except in the presence of documented infected necrosis, or in patients with necrotizing pancreatitis who are not improving clinically without antibiotic use. Antibiotics known to penetrate necrotic tissue (such as carbapenems, quinolones and metronidazole) should be used in management of infected pancreatic necrosis as these may delay surgical intervention and decrease morbidity and mortality. Instead antiprotease or antioxidants are not recommended in the management of acute pancreatitis in children [15].

2.4.2 Nutritional strategy

In severe pancreatitis an earlier oral re-feeding reduces the incidence of infections and contributes to a shorter hospitalization. Serum pancreatic enzymes' level tips the balance in the enteral feeding strategy. If serum amylase and lipase are decreasing liquid intake can be started, according with clinical conditions, while if they are minor than two times the upper normal values, an hypolipidic diet should be considered [13].

2.4.3 Endoscopic and surgical treatment

Undoubtedly anatomic abnormalities are an indication for surgery while ampulla of Vater anomalies or pancreatic divisum may be eligible for an endoscopic sphincterotomy. In patients with infected necrosis of the pancreatic gland a necrosectomy is mandatory in case of worsening clinical conditions and unresponsiveness to therapeutic measures. However this procedure (percutaneous, endoscopic or laparoscopic necrosectomy) has an high mortality rate and should be performed in hemodynamically stable patients.

Pancreatic pseudocysts are cysts that develop due to injury of the pancreatic duct and extravasation of fluid. These occur 4 weeks or later after the onset of pancreatitis. Treatment is indicated for pseudocysts if their size does not decrease, if they are accompanied by abdominal pain, or if there are complications of infection or hemorrhage. Whereas endoscopic ultrasound-guided transgastric drainage can safely be considered in case of growing pancreatic pseudocysts or in case of hemorrhagic complications [13].

3. Acute recurrent pancreatitis

Approximately 10–20% of pediatric patients experience recurrent episodes of acute pancreatitis beneath which it is possible to identify an idiopathic or structural etiology. ARP may evolve in the chronic form that is clinically indistinguishable from acute pancreatitis in children [16].

3.1 Etiology

Risk factors that predispose to ARP can be categorized according the following frequency in: genetic, obstructive, metabolic and autoimmune [17]. However the etiology of ARP remains unexplained in 30% of cases and can be classified as "idiopathic" is used.

3.1.1 Genetic causes

Genetic conditions that predispose to recurrent episodes of pancreatitis are the cystic fibrosis transmembrane conductance regulator-gene (CFTR-gene), PRSS1-gene and SPINK1-gene mutations.

CFTR-gene mutations occur in about 5% of Western populations and cause an altered function of the product of this gene with a defect in the transmembrane epithelial chloride ion transfer. This dysregulation affects different organs including the pancreas and results in an abnormal production of viscous exocrine secretions that lead to ductal obstructions. Mutations in the cationic trypsinogen gene (**PRSS1-gene**) have been matched in patients with hereditary pancreatitis. The pancreas is unable to contrast an excessive trypsin activation because of the lack of protective mechanism predisposing patients to recurrent episodes of pancreatitis in childhood.

SPINK1-gene mutations predispose to the development pancreatitis and involve the serine protease inhibitor Kazal type I gene (SPINK1). This mutation results in a defect of the protective action in the pancreas mediated by SPINK1 protein that represents a feedback inhibitor of trypsin activation. Approximately 16–23% of patients with idiopathic pancreatitis have SPINK1 mutations instead [18].

3.1.2 Anatomical anomalies

Pancreas divisum is the most frequent anatomical variant and has an incidence near to 12% in general population. As a result of this incomplete fusion of the ventral and dorsal ducts pancreatic juices cause ductal hypertension. Patients may experience recurrent pain after food intake, an alteration in serum content of pancreatic enzymes, or acute recurrent pancreatitis. Annular pancreas is another anatomical variant that may be related with duodenal or biliary obstructive symptoms. Ductal abnormalities such as a common pancreatico-biliary channel may determine a bile or pancreatic juices reflux and can be diagnosed with ERCP. Sphincter of Oddi dysfunction (SOD) is another factor predisposing to ARP and is probably the most common cause of the idiopathic form. This dysfunction includes two clinical forms: SO increased basal pressure related to a structural fibrotic alteration of the sphincter and SO dyskinesia, caused by sphincter hypertone [19].

3.1.3 Metabolic disorders

Toxic and metabolic factors such as hypercalcemia, hypertriglyceridemia, diabetes, porphyria and Wilson's disease can predispose to the development of acute recurrent episodes of pancreatitis as well as medications (i.e., azathioprine and 6-mercaptopurine) [17].

3.1.4 Autoimmune disorders

Autoimmune pancreatitis is an increasingly recognized disease entity associated with hypergammaglobulinemia. High serum levels of IgG4 are suggestive of AIP in adults while just 22% of pediatric patients have immunoglobulin levels above the upper limits of normal [19]. AIP can be classified into two types: type one lymphoplasmacytic sclerosing pancreatitis and type two idiopathic duct-centric pancreatitis. The latter form seems to be more frequent in children and it is associated with inflammatory bowel syndrome. Anyway this distinctive type of pancreatitis is responsive to corticosteroid therapy.

3.2 Clinical features and diagnosis

ARP can be defined as two or more episodes of acute pancreatitis occurring with complete resolution of symptoms in between (>1 month between two episodes) or normalization of pancreatic enzymes serum levels in the time interval, with not detected radiological signs of chronic pancreatitis. ARP should be considered in the diagnostic process of children with a positive anamnesis for recurrent gastroenteritis with vomiting, epigastric pain, or irritable bowel syndrome. An early identification of the underlying etiology may lead to a complete resolution of the disease [18].

The most common risk factors in childhood are genetic mutations so gene testing is mandatory and a chloride sweat test is helpful to diagnose a CF (cystic fibrosis).

The patient's anamnesis and standard laboratory tests, trans-abdominal ultrasound, MRCP, and CT scan can easily detect the causes of recurrent pancreatitis in about 70% of cases. The remaining 30% of patients should have further investigations such as genetic testing, MRCP (magnetic resonance cholangiopancreatography), that provides the potential to delineate ductal anatomy without the risks of contrast injection, EUS (Endoscopic UltraSonography) and ERCP, that represents the most accurate imaging to define the pancreas anatomy. Genetic and autoimmune pancreatitis can be diagnosed by sequencing CFTR or SPINK1/PRSS1 gene mutations and IgG4.

3.3 Treatment

Therapeutic approach to recurrent pancreatitis associated with pancreas divisum is based on endoscopic and surgical procedures. Both strategies are effective in 70–90% so the former therapy is preferred. Surgery may include accessory duct sphincteroplasty alone or in combination with major sphincteroplasty and septoplasty. Patients with distal ductal obstruction or ductal ectasia may take advantage from pancreaticojejunostomy [20]. Annular pancreas is another congenital alateration of the pancreatic ductal system and surgical resection represents the preferential treatment. Recurrent pancreatitis associated with the CFTR-gene mutation of hereditary pancreatitis may be prevented by endoscopic pancreatic sphincterotomy reducing intraductal hypertension.

Furthermore, in last years, many efforts have been made to identify a novel therapy for lipoprotein lipase deficiency (LPLD), a genetic disease causing chylomicronemia and an increased risk for developing acute and recurrent pancreatitis. Thus alipogene tiparvovec (Glybera) gene therapy has definitely proven to be effective in reducing frequency and severity of pancreatitis events [21].

4. Chronic pancreatitis

Pediatric chronic pancreatitis is unusual and the incidence increases with age (0.5 per 100,000 in young adults) but this condition presents a progressive behavior and is poorly responsive to therapy.

Chronic pancreatitis has been defined as a persistent inflammatory injury of the pancreas characterized by irreversible architectural changes that cause pain and/or irreversible loss of function [22].

4.1 Etiology

As mentioned above genetic mutations are the most common causative factors for pancreatitis in children despite other risk factors may be brought into play as the TIGAR-O classification system well explained and categorized according to toxic-metabolic causes, idiopathic, genetic, autoimmune and obstructive chronic pancreatitis [23]. Within the last years, multiple studies have reported rates of genetic mutations associated with pancreatitis, involving CFTR, SPINK1 and PRSS1 genes, from 36 to 73%. So future perspectives will certainly focus on a personalized medicine approach in order to define a more specific and targeted treatment. Cationic trypsinogen PRSS1 is the gene most frequently involved in the evolution to the end stage of chronic pancreatitis. Near to 80% of individuals with either the R122H or N29I gain of function mutation develop at least one episode of acute pancreatitis and half of clinically affected individuals with either the R122H or N29I mutation will evolve to chronic pancreatitis.

Moreover pancreas divisum represents an obstructive cofactor in the development of chronic involutional changes of the pancreatic gland.

4.2 Pathology

Parenchymal fibrosis, with loss of acinar cells, results in exocrine pancreatic insufficiency (EPI) as a late stage of the disease and needs to be treated with pancreatic enzyme replacement therapies. Then normal acini are replaced by fibroblasts and lymphocytic infiltration. Furthermore, progressively endocrine cells are damaged too resulting in diabetes mellitus (DM) that often occurs post chronic pancreatitis [23].

4.3 Diagnosis

According with INSPPIRE data the definition of chronic pediatric pancreatitis depends upon one of the following: (1) abdominal pain and imaging findings that can suggest a chronic pancreatic damage; (2) evidence of exocrine pancreatic insufficiency with maldigestions symptoms and diagnostic imaging suggestive for pancreatic damage; (3) evidence of pancreatic islets dysfunction and imaging findings that can suggest the presence of a pancreatic damage; or (4) a surgical or pancreatic biopsy demonstrating pathological features compatible with chronic pancreatitis [24].

4.3.1 Imaging findings

The most commonly found radiographic signs of chronic pancreatitis in children are represented by ductal anomalies and pancreatic gland atrophy. Unlike the adult form, pancreatic calcifications are not detected in childhood chronic pancreatitis.

To reduce the exposure to ionizing radiation MRI/MRCP and ultrasound (US) are preferred. ERCP, as in adults, can be considered for procedures such as stone removal or stricture dilation [23].

4.3.2 Pancreatic function tests

Altered pancreatic function tests are diagnostic of chronic pancreatitis but also are detected in case of other clinical conditions such as pancreatic agenesis or resection, intestinal atrophy, kwashiorkor and gastrinoma. We also have to consider mild or moderate forms of chronic pancreatitis in case of normal tests. Exocrine pancreatic function can be assessed by direct or indirect evaluations. Direct tests pancreatic such as the secretin-cholecystokinin test have the highest sensitivity and specificity but at the same time they are inadequate for routine clinical practice in pediatric population. On the other hand indirect tests are noninvasive and routinely used. Indirect pancreatic function test can be divided in three main groups:

1. Analysis of the hydrolyzed products of pancreatic enzymes' activity detectable in urine and serum (NBT-PABA test, pancreolauryl test);

2. Assessment of undigested and unabsorbed food components in feces (fecal fat excretion and fecal fat concentration);

3. Dosage of pancreatic enzymes in the serum (amylase, isoamylase, lipase, trypsinogen, elastase-1) or stool (chymotrypsin, lipase, elastase-1).

Fecal elastase-1 (FE1) is the most sensitive test in the evaluation of exocrine pancreatic function in chronic pancreatitis [25].

Fecal elastase-1 is a proteolytic pancreatic enzyme that is not degraded during its passage through the gastrointestinal tract. Analysis of FE1 is simple and practical to be managed but it may be compromised in case of diarrhea, with an associated risk of falsely low FE1 concentration [26].

4.3.3 Biopsy

A pancreatic EUS-guided biopsy may represent the gold standard for the diagnosis of chronic pancreatitis but it is not widely available.

And besides some etiologies of chronic pancreatitis, such as autoimmune or hereditary pancreatitis, need multiple biopsies to be diagnostic. At histological examination irregular fibrosis can be seen while intralobular fibrosis alone is not specific for chronic pancreatitis [22].

4.4 Treatment

Both the stage and etiology of CP influence its management. With disease progression, chronic pain management and treatment of pancreatic insufficiency or diabetes are required. Acetaminophen may be effective in the early stages, but therapy generally advances to narcotics. Pancreatic enzyme supplements and antioxidant therapy (selenium, ascorbic acid, b-carotene, a-tocopherol, and methionine) are prescribed frequently in this setting. Endoscopic treatment for CP should be considered only when ductal strictures or pancreatic duct calculi are present or for symptomatic pseudocysts. Surgical treatment is still indicated in selected patients when conservative treatment failed. Localized disease can be treated with partial pancreatic resection (i.e., in case of a pancreatic inflammatory head mass) while radical pancreatectomy with islet cell autotransplant is currently offered to patients who have genetic causes of pancreatitis (as we'll describe in the next section). A longitudinal pancreaticojejunostomy (known as modified Puestow procedure) can be definitely avoided. Although many patients have pain relief, a number of patients continue to have pain. In up to 20% of adults, the pain is as intense as it was before the resection. Preadolescents are more likely to be insulin-independent than older children and adults. Thus time to surgical procedure is fundamental to avoid a progressive decrease in islet cell yield. Pancreatic insufficiency is treated with pancreatic enzyme replacement therapy. The final goal is to restore digestive function and maintain weight gain.

4.4.1 Total pancreatectomy with islet autotransplantation (TPIAT)

Children with chronic pancreatitis who suffer recurrent severe episodes of abdominal pain, chronic use of analgesics (opioids) and frequent hospitalizations may benefit from TPIAT, in order to improve their quality of life. A multidisciplinary team including gastroenterologists, endocrinologists, surgeons, anesthesiologists, psychologists, radiologists and nutritionists guides the selection of these patients.

Thus the procedure consists in a demolitive operative phase, followed by a reconstructive one that includes an hepaticojejunostomy plus gastrojejunostomy or a duodenojejunostomy and the autotransplantation of islets via the portal vein.

Osmotic, mechanical or hypoxia damage of islets should be considered, especially in the pre-engraftment phase and the risk of developing diabetes mellitus must be accepted by families.

Anyway pain resolution, independence from analgesics and significant improvement in quality of life has been reported in the majority of children with CP following TPIAT, and glycemic control is managed without difficulty [24, 27].

5. Conclusions

The incidence of acute pancreatitis is increasing in children and it should be considered as part of differential diagnosis in case of abdominal pain. The etiology of acute pancreatitis in this subpopulation is related to several conditions and risk factors, such as drugs, obesity, infections, trauma and anatomic abnormalities but genetic predisposition represents the master causative factor.

Rapid and accurate assessment of severity is useful for selecting an appropriate initial treatment and predicting the prognosis. The International Study Group for Pediatric Pancreatitis: In Search for a Cure (INSPPIRE) focused on ARP and CP in pediatrics and we can delineate more accurately clinical presentations, risk factors and natural history of pediatric pancreatitis to define a more appropriate therapeutic strategy, often considering that a children is not a small adult.

Author details

Stefano Valabrega[1*], Laura Bersigotti[1], Laura Antolino[1], Paolo Aurello[1],
Federico Tomassini[1], P. Valabrega[3], S. Amato[1], Francesco D' Angelo[1], Luciano Izzo[2]
and Salvatore Caterino[1]

1 Department of Surgical and Medical Sciences, Sapienza University of Rome, Italy

2 Department of Surgery "P. Valdoni", Sapienza University of Rome, Italy

3 Pediatric Division, Vevey Hospital, Switzerland

*Address all correspondence to: stefano.valabrega@uniroma1.it

IntechOpen

References

[1] Pohl JF et al. Pediatric pancreatitis. Current Opinion in Gastroenterology. 2015

[2] Rawla P et al. Review of infectious etiology of acute pancreatitis. Gastroenterology Research. 2017

[3] Suzuki M et al. Acute pancreatitis in children and adolescents. World Journal of Gastrointestinal Pathophysiology. 2014

[4] Bai HX et al. Novel characterization of drug-associated pancreatitis in children. Journal of Pediatric Gastroenterology and Nutrition. 2011

[5] Stefanovic M et al. Acute pancreatitis as a complication of childhood cancer treatment. Cancer Medicine. 2016

[6] Hong MJ et al. Pancreatic laceration in a pediatric patient: An unexpected diagnosis. Case Reports in Pediatrics. 2017

[7] Shrinat A et al. Pediatric pancreatitis. Pediatrics in Review. 2013

[8] Cappel MS et al. Acute pancreatitis: Etiology, clinical presentation, diagnosis and therapy. The Medical Clinics of North America. 2008

[9] Grzybowska-Chlebowczyk U et al. Acute pancreatitis in children. Gastroenterology Review. 2018

[10] Shukela-Udawatta M et al. An update on pediatric pancreatitis. Pediatric Annals. 2017

[11] Restrepo R et al. Acute pancreatitis in pediatric patients: Demographicsβ, etiology and diagnostic imaging. American Journal of Roentgenology. 2016

[12] Lautz TB et al. Acute pancreatitis in children: Spectrum of disease and predictors of severity. Journal of Pediatric Surgery. 2011

[13] Suzuky M et al. Scoring system for the prediction of severe acute pancreatitis in children. Pediatrics International. 2014

[14] Chadley Thabet F et al. Intra-abdominal hypertension and abdominal compartment syndrome in pediatrics. A review. Journal of Critical Care. 2017

[15] Abu-El-Haija M et al. Management of acute pancreatitis in the pediatric population: A clinical report from the north American society for pediatric gastroenterology, hepatology and nutrition pancreas committee. Journal of Pediatric Gastroenterology and Nutrition. 2018

[16] Lucidi V et al. The etiology of acute recurrent pancreatitis in children: A challenge for pediatricians. Pancreas. 2011

[17] Kumar S et al. Risk factors associated with pediatric acute recurrent and chronic pancreatitis lessons from insppire. JAMA Pediatrics. 2016

[18] Testoni PA et al. Acute recurrent pancreatitis: Etiopathogenesis, diagnosis and treatment. World Journal of Gastroenterology. 2014

[19] Sheen I et al. Autoimmune pancreatitis in children: Characteristic features, diagnosis and management. The American Journal of Gastroenterology. 2017

[20] Wallace W, Neblett III, et al. Surgical management of recurrent pancreatitis in children with pancreas divisum. Annals of Surgery. 2000

[21] Gaudet D et al. Long-term retrospective analysis of gene therapy with alipogene tiparvovec and its effect on lipoprotein lipase deficiency-induced pancreatitis. Human Gene Therapy. 2016

[22] Etemad B et al. Chronic pancreatitis: Diagnosis, classification, and new genetic developments. Gastroenterology. 2001

[23] Abu-El-Haija M et al. Pediatric chronic pancreatitis: Updates in the 21st century. Pancreatology. 2018

[24] Schwarzenberg SJ et al. Pediatric chronic pancreatitis is associated with genetic risk factors and substantial disease burden. The Journal of Pediatrics. 2015

[25] Walkowiak J et al. Indirect pancreatic function tests in children. Journal of Pediatric Gastroenterology and Nutrition. 2005

[26] Williams N et al. The role, yield and cost of paediatric faecal elastase-1 testing. Pancreatology. 2016

[27] Weber T et al. Operative management of chronic pancreatitis in children. Archives of Surgery. 2001

www.ingramcontent.com/pod-product-compliance
Lightning Source LLC
Chambersburg PA
CBHW081236190326
41458CB00016B/5807